THE
BLOOD SUGAR
BALANCING
HANDBOOK

....

Simple Recipes, Proven Methods, and Practical Strategies for Improving Glucose Levels for Non-Diabetics

....

Autumn Enloe,
MS, RD, LD

Published by:
Ulysses Press
PO Box 3440
Berkeley, CA 94703
www.ulyssespress.com

ISBN: 978-1-64604-736-9
Library of Congress Control Number: 2024934570

Printed in the United States
10 9 8 7 6 5 4 3 2 1

Acquisitions editor: Claire Sielaff
Managing editor: Claire Chun
Editor: Sherian Brown
Proofreader: Laurie Dunne
Front cover design: Ashley Prine
Artwork: cover and part opening pages © Alexandra Anschiz/shutterstock.com;
      page 40 © Anastasiia Usenko/shutterstock.com; page 59 © Safety System
      /shutterstock.com
Layout: Winnie Liu

CONTENTS

Introduction   1

PART 1: THE IMPORTANCE OF BLOOD SUGAR   3

CHAPTER 1: What Is Blood Sugar?   4

CHAPTER 2: Why Your Blood Sugar Is a Foundational Piece of Your Health   7

CHAPTER 3: Assessing Your Blood Sugar   15

PART 2: WHAT YOU CAN DO TO OPTIMIZE YOUR BLOOD SUGAR WITH NUTRITION   19

CHAPTER 4: Getting Off the Blood Sugar Roller Coaster   20

CHAPTER 5: Balancing Your Plate with Protein, Carbohydrates, and Fats   26

CHAPTER 6: The Glycemic Index of Foods   43

CHAPTER 7: The Magic of Vitamins and Minerals   48

CHAPTER 8: What About Sugar?   55

CHAPTER 9: Breakfast and Blood Sugars   63

CHAPTER 10: Practicing Mindful Eating   67

CHAPTER 11: All About Hydration   72

CHAPTER 12: Navigating Nutrition Labels and Grocery Shopping   77

CHAPTER 13: Mastering Meal Prep   82

PART 3: **LOOKING AT THE BIG PICTURE OF HEALTH**   87

CHAPTER 14: The Link Between Cortisol and Blood Sugar   88

CHAPTER 15: What's Your Gut Have to Do With It?   98

CHAPTER 16: Movement Is Medicine   104

CHAPTER 17: The Importance of Zzz's for Balanced
Blood Sugars   109

CHAPTER 18: Are There Supplements to Help Improve
Blood Sugar?   114

CHAPTER 19: Putting It All Together   117

Final Thoughts   122

PART 4: **RECIPES**   124

Breakfast   126

Main Dishes   133

Salads   141

Sides and Snacks   145

Beverages   150

Bibliography   153

Acknowledgments   162

About the Author   164

INTRODUCTION

As a registered dietitian, I get asked a lot of nutrition questions like, "What should I eat to lose weight?" or "How can I improve my energy?" or "I'm addicted to sugar—how do I stop craving it all the time?"

No matter what the question is, nine times out of ten it's related to a blood sugar issue.

This is a topic I talk about with every client no matter what their health goal is, because it's the foundation for your health. Literally.

My passion for blood sugar comes from both personal and professional experience. I've struggled with an imbalance in blood sugar levels, feeling like I was always "hangry" and wanting to snack all the time despite "*doing all the right things.*" I've also become more intrigued with this topic after working one-on-one with clients over the past decade and seeing the impact it has on long-term health.

I've seen blood sugar regulation change lives. I've had clients who were able to get off medications they thought they would have to stay on for the rest of their lives, clients who were finally losing weight without going on a diet or counting a single calorie, and clients who have reported so much more energy, less sugar cravings, and better sleep by following the blood sugar tips and strategies you'll learn in this book.

Many clients are surprised when I bring up blood sugar because it's a topic that is mainly discussed only if you've been diagnosed with prediabetes or diabetes. After I explain that it plays a key role in everything from your cravings to energy to hormone and metabolic health, it clicks.

Although this book is focused on preventative health and geared toward non-diabetes, it's still beneficial if you or someone you know has a prediabetes or diabetes diagnosis. You can incorporate the same concepts in this book while working with your healthcare provider.

Note: this isn't a quick-fix diet program. This is your go-to resource for all things related to blood sugar (and so much more!). We'll go through everything from how to balance your meals and snacks to stay full longer and become more energized, how to support digestion so you can absorb the nutrients from your food more effectively, and how to crush your sugar cravings so you can stop relying on willpower, to optimizing your blood sugars with nonstressful exercise and better-quality sleep. It's filled with simple strategies you can implement for years and years to come.

I've included some reflection questions throughout this book, as well as some "quick tips" to help you absorb the information better. It is not intended to replace medical advice but to be a resource to assist you with your health right now and prevent health complications in the future. As with any new health change, focus on keeping it simple and realistic.

Alright, ready to get started? Let's go.

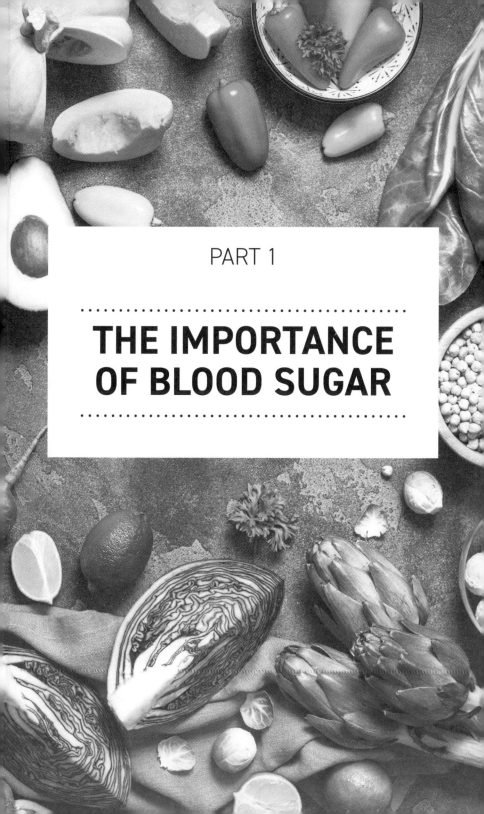

PART 1

THE IMPORTANCE OF BLOOD SUGAR

WHAT IS BLOOD SUGAR?

"You cannot always control what goes on outside, but you can always control what goes on inside."

—Wayne Dyer

"I'm not diabetic. I don't need to worry about my blood sugar."

I was doing an assessment with my new client Sarah and asking about any lab work she'd had done, including her blood sugar labs. She showed me the information she recently received from her doctor, and I asked about labs like her hemoglobin A1C (the average blood sugar for three months) and fasting glucose. She told me she wasn't diabetic, so she didn't think she needed to worry about getting lab work done on her blood sugar. Her doctor didn't bring it up either.

Although blood sugar is a huge focus for those who are diagnosed with prediabetes or diabetes, everyone should be paying attention to blood sugar levels from a prevention standpoint. With almost thirty million Americans diagnosed with diabetes, almost nine million individuals are left undiagnosed (American Diabetes Association 2023).

Our current healthcare system is set up to treat you *when* you get a diagnosis, versus focusing on *preventing* the diagnosis from even occurring. Most people are walking around stressed, exhausted, and sick because our environment and healthcare system are not focused on prevention. Oftentimes, a health concern will trigger action (like a diet change or new medication), but what if you could prevent that health concern from happening in the first place? If more people focused on their blood sugar levels from a preventative standpoint, I can only imagine how many Americans might never get the *"You have diabetes"* diagnosis in the first place.

Paying attention to your blood sugars can not just help prevent health complications in the future; it can also help with many struggles you may be experiencing now. Issues like fatigue, sugar cravings, inflammation, weight loss resistance, hot flashes or night sweats, PMS (premenstrual syndrome) symptoms, hormonal acne, brain fog, bloating, irritability, and anxiety have all been tied to blood sugar levels.

SO, WHAT IS BLOOD SUGAR AND WHY IS IT SUCH A BIG DEAL?

Say you're munching on a donut or having a banana for a snack. No matter what the source of carbohydrate is, the body breaks down the carbohydrates into a sugar called *glucose.* This is the body's favorite source of fuel. Lab tests (like a fasting glucose, for example) will look at the blood glucose levels as a way to measure the amount of sugar in the body at a single moment. Please note, in this book, *blood sugar* and *blood glucose* are terms that are used interchangeably.

So what does the body do with all that broken-down glucose? The body regulates blood glucose levels by releasing a hormone called *insulin* from the pancreas to bring the glucose from the bloodstream into the cells to be used for energy. Insulin is a fat-storage hormone, and chronic high levels of insulin can increase the risk for type 2 diabetes, fatigue, faster aging, weight gain, and hormone imbalances. Carbohydrates influence the ebb and flow of insulin, but so do things like the balance of macronutrients at a meal, the timing and how you're eating your meals, your daily movement, stress levels, and sleep habits, just to name a few.

After eating, blood glucose levels rise, and how quickly or slowly your blood glucose levels increase is based on the types of foods you're consuming. For example, eating foods high in sugar or refined carbohydrates will cause a larger and quicker blood glucose spike compared to foods high in fiber.

The balance of your meals and snacks are also critical. For example, eating carbohydrates alone can cause a higher spike in blood glucose, but if you pair that carbohydrate with a protein source, the protein can act as a buffer and prevent such a large spike from happening.

Glucose is used for a quick source of energy for the body, and if you consume more than your body needs, the extra glucose will get stored in your liver, muscles, and fat tissues for later use. Your blood sugar levels can either be a helpful tool for improving areas like metabolic and hormone health, brain function, energy, sleep, and digestion, or it can impact those areas in a negative way if levels aren't balanced. That's why managing and optimizing your blood sugar is key for optimal health. We'll get into balancing your plate better for optimal blood sugar levels in Chapter 5, but for now, know that you have the power to change your health with the foods you're eating every single day. This book is here to show you how.

In my work as a registered dietitian, I've seen the powerful impact that diet and lifestyle habits can have on blood glucose levels. I've seen clients reverse a diabetes diagnosis, get off medications, and feel healthier and more energetic than they had twenty years ago. I've seen clients no longer have brain fog or sugar cravings and lose weight without counting a single calorie. Their stories can be your story too, because the first thing they all prioritized was their blood sugar balance. Yes, blood sugar is a key marker for health for those with prediabetes or diabetes, but it's also essential for non-diabetics as well.

Let's dig deeper into this in the next chapter.

> **Quick tip:** Focusing on regulating your blood sugar can help improve energy levels, moods, hormones, metabolism, sleep, and more.

WHY YOUR BLOOD SUGAR IS A FOUNDATIONAL PIECE OF YOUR HEALTH

"What most people don't realize is that food is not just calories; it's information. It actually contains messages that communicate to every cell in the body."

—Dr. Mark Hyman

Balancing blood sugar is one of the foundational pieces I work on with every single client, no matter what their health goal is. Want to lose weight and get stronger? Have more energy? Crush your sugar cravings? Have better thyroid health? Stop feeling bloated all the time? Improve conditions like PCOS? Have healthy, pain-free periods? Sleep better at night? Age gracefully? Want to be able to think better at work and remember what you ate an hour ago? It all starts with supporting your blood sugar.

Think about it like this: focusing on your health without paying attention to blood sugar is like trying to drive your car without putting any gas in it. You just can't do it. Now maybe you're wondering why this topic isn't talked about very often, and truthfully I'm just as curious as you. There's way too much focus on calories or a lack of willpower and not enough on the quality and composition of meals . . . until now.

Let's dive into how blood sugar impacts several areas of health.

BLOOD SUGAR AND ENERGY

One of the most common complaints I hear from clients is the lack of energy they feel. Unfortunately, America is not set up like Europe where we can take a two-hour lunch break and nap midday. So, we push through. We grab more coffee or a candy bar to give us an energy boost, eat a huge dinner at night because we're starving, and scroll on our phone before bed as our way to "relax." No wonder we're exhausted.

Although many factors can contribute to low energy, one of the main culprits for low energy is an imbalance in blood sugar. That's because glucose is the main source of energy for the body. When blood glucose levels get too low, your energy will also get low. This is often why people experience the afternoon slump, the feeling of fatigue around two or three o'clock in the afternoon. Their blood sugar levels have dropped since lunch, possibly from not eating enough earlier in the day, or an imbalance in macronutrients at their meals. That's why focusing on eating three balanced, nutrient-dense meals, and including a balanced snack if needed, can help support stable, balanced blood sugars and keep energy levels up.

Quick blood sugar spikes and drops can also influence energy levels. For example, having a high-carb breakfast that doesn't contain much protein or nourishing fat (like a bagel with cream cheese and some fruit) will cause blood glucose levels to increase quickly, and then drop quickly. Many people are riding this blood sugar roller-coaster ride all day long, which is leaving them feeling exhausted. I'll talk more about the blood sugar roller coaster soon.

BLOOD SUGAR AND WEIGHT

Although we've been told to eat less and move more for weight loss, there's so much more to it than that. Of course exercise is key for optimal health, but simply focusing on cutting calories is not always the answer. Our health (and weight) is much more than a simple math equation of calories in, calories out. In fact, if you aren't eating enough nutrient-dense foods for your body to keep your organs healthy, brain fueled, and muscles strong, it can actually slow down your metabolism. Yes, the average American consumes more calories (about 20 percent) than even twenty years ago, but oftentimes those calories are low-nutrient calories. So even if someone is consuming enough calories for what their body needs, those calories aren't able to be used in ways that the body needs. It's like having plants at home that you never water. Sure, they may do okay for a short time, but eventually the leaves become brown and wilted. The types of foods you're eating, your consistency with how often you eat, and improving blood sugar levels will have the greatest impact on your weight. For example, studies have shown eating three consistent meals throughout the day has the greatest impact on weight, type 2 diabetes, and cardiovascular disease (Manoogian et al. 2018). Likewise, another study found that improving blood sugar levels and insulin sensitivity resulted in a greater chance of weight loss (Kong et al. 2020). Prioritizing balanced and consistent meals to optimize blood sugar and fuel your metabolism will be more beneficial for reaching your healthiest weight than simply focusing on calories alone.

BLOOD SUGAR AND DIGESTION

"After the kids go to bed, I go to my pantry, and I just can't stop eating." This was one of my clients who was a busy working mom. She came to me with years of struggling with bloating despite not eating much during her day. She barely ate anything for breakfast and would just have a couple bites of food at lunch due to feeling rushed at work. She would come home and eat her largest meal of the day in the evening and then raid the pantry after the kids fell asleep because she was still starving. This is a common scenario I see with clients, and one that can also be an easy fix. Digestive issues like bloating, heartburn, gas, constipation, or diarrhea can be a result of some type of sensitivity to a particular food or a lack of digestive enzymes to break down the food properly. They can also occur from an imbalance in blood sugars, like they did for this client. Let me explain.

When a person skips meals, or doesn't eat enough at a meal, it increases the chances of overeating later on (which was the case for my client). When this happens, our digestion has to work overtime, and emptying of the stomach slows down, leading to symptoms like bloating, stomach pain, or indigestion. Also, it's easy to eat quickly when you're really hungry, which contributes to even more digestive issues. Instead, eating three balanced meals consistently each day is a lot easier for your digestive system to do the job it's designed to do.

On the flip side, grazing all day can also contribute to digestive issues. It takes about three hours for your food to go from the stomach to the small intestine where it breaks down and absorbs the food. If you're constantly snacking on food throughout the day, your digestive system doesn't have the opportunity to rest. Make sure to give your digestive system a break throughout the day by allowing a three(ish)-hour window between any meal or snack.

We'll dive deeper into digestion in Chapter 15.

BLOOD SUGAR AND HORMONE HEALTH

Your blood sugar is linked to several hormones, including insulin, estrogen, the appetite hormones ghrelin and leptin, cortisol, growth hormone, and the GLP-1 hormone.

Insulin is one of the hormones most influenced by blood sugar levels. As discussed in Chapter 1, insulin is a fat-storage hormone. Too much insulin can lead to cells in the body becoming desensitized (meaning they won't open the door when insulin is knocking because the party is full), and it increases the risk for developing type 2 diabetes, cardiovascular disease, hypertension, fatty liver disease, fatigue, and weight gain. Elevated levels can also increase testosterone in women and lead to facial hair or acne, and increase the risk for Polycystic ovary syndrome (PCOS), along with lowering sex hormone-binding globulin (SHBG) and contribute to PMS symptoms and heavy periods.

Blood sugars are also associated with your appetite hormones, ghrelin and leptin. Ghrelin is the hunger hormone that sends a signal to your brain when the stomach is empty and it's time to eat. Leptin, on the other hand, prevents hunger and helps regulate energy balance so you don't feel hungry all the time. Not only does blood sugar regulation improve insulin levels, it also supports leptin levels. This means that you stay full longer and can burn your calories more effectively.

Another area where blood sugars impact hormones is related to the thyroid hormones, which play a key role in energy and metabolic health. Blood sugar and the thyroid work interchangeably. For example, thyroid hormones are essential for carbohydrate metabolism, and if a person has hypothyroidism (where the thyroid isn't producing enough thyroid hormone) insulin doesn't work as well in the body and can lead to low blood sugar levels. Likewise, not eating enough carbohydrates, or having consistent low blood sugar levels, can decrease the thyroid's ability to produce a healthy balance of thyroid hormones. We'll talk more about carbohydrates in Chapter 5, but for now, know that carbohydrates are essential for optimal thyroid health.

Lastly, blood sugar is also linked to the GLP-1 hormone (glucagon-like peptide) as well. GLP-1 hormone is considered an "anti-hunger" hormone that helps regulate digestion, appetite, and blood sugar levels by stimulating the release of insulin. Prioritizing balancing your meals with all the macronutrients, especially with protein and fiber-rich carbohydrates, can help stimulate GLP-1 secretion (Hira et al. 2021).

BLOOD SUGAR AND STRESS

You've probably heard about cortisol, the stress hormone, before. Although some stress can be beneficial for the body, too much isn't a great thing and can lead to long-term health consequences. When it comes to your blood sugars, elevated cortisol also contributes to a higher amount of insulin being secreted. Remember how too much insulin isn't a great thing because it can increase your risk for health issues like weight gain (especially around the abdomen) and type 2 diabetes? Stress has a significant impact on metabolic health, and issues with blood sugar can be triggered by stress in the body. We'll talk more about stress in Chapter 14, but for now, know that managing stress is something that is not only critical for optimal blood sugars but also for your health long-term.

I've seen countless times the impact stress can have on health goals. Sure, bubble baths or getting massages can be helpful for reducing stress in the body, but there's so much that can be done on a daily basis to improve stress levels in the body, and it starts with balancing your blood sugar.

BLOOD SUGAR AND HEART HEALTH

Heart disease is the leading cause of death for both men and women, and your blood sugars can impact that risk.

Elevated blood sugar levels can cause the blood vessels and nerves that control the heart to become damaged. That's one reason why individuals with diabetes are more likely to have other conditions that increase the risk for heart disease, like elevated triglyceride levels or high low-density lipoprotein (LDL), as well as high blood pressure (Centers for Disease Control and Prevention 2022). If you're looking to improve your lipid panel and lower your risk for heart disease, prioritizing blood sugar balance is the first place to start.

BLOOD SUGAR AND CRAVINGS

Clients often tell me they feel like they're a sugar addict. Not surprising, considering the average person eats about sixty pounds of sugar each year. If you've ever wondered how someone can keep Oreo cookies in their cupboard without devouring the entire package in one sitting, know you're not alone.

Sugar cravings are a huge problem for many people, and simply relying on willpower to get you through isn't the answer. So what helps reduce sugar cravings? You guessed it—blood sugar regulation. That's because when blood glucose levels get low, your body protects you by telling you it needs more sugar to raise it back up. So whether your blood sugar is on a roller-coaster ride with large spikes and drops during the day, or you have continuous low blood sugar by not eating enough calories for what your body needs, you'll naturally crave more sugar during the day because your body is trying to balance itself out.

What about chronic high blood sugar? That can trigger sugar cravings as well. In fact, the higher your blood sugar level goes up, the louder your cravings can get. Unfortunately, with all the additives and sugars found in the foods today, as well as the constant access to food wherever we go, many people are riding on this crazy roller-coaster ride all day long.

It's pretty difficult to find packaged foods without added sugar. That favored coffee drink you're getting from the drive-thru in the morning, the granola bar you have for a snack, or the ketchup you top your burger with all contains added sugar. The more sugar we consume, the more we tend to crave it. So when blood sugar levels become more supported by focusing on nutrient-dense whole foods, sugar cravings can start to decrease.

I hope you're noticing the power that a healthy blood sugar level can have on your health, not just immediately but also long-term. So how can you tell if your blood sugar is in a healthy range? Let me walk you through that in the next chapter.

But first, I encourage you to do some reflection on your current health status.

REFLECTION

1. *List your current health struggles and rate them on a scale of 1–10 (10 being the most severe and 1 meaning it hardly impacts you at all).*

----

2. *Next, if you had a magic wand and could magically make those health struggles disappear, how would your life change? What could you do that you aren't able to do now? How would you look and feel?*

> **Quick Tip:** Focus on blood sugar support + the quality
> of your food over the calories in it.

CHAPTER 3

ASSESSING YOUR BLOOD SUGAR

"Half the costs of illness are wasted on conditions that could be prevented."

—Dr. Joseph Pizzorno

"I feel like I'm constantly hungry and thinking about food all day." This is what my client Katie told me when I first met with her. These were red flags that her body was not getting enough nourishing calories and her blood sugar needed support. I explained to her how our bodies are like cars—they need fuel to get us where we need them to go. You wouldn't expect to go on a road trip with an empty tank of gas, right? Yet we often expect our bodies to do everything we want them to do without even filling the tank well enough. Before long, we're stuck on the side of the highway calling roadside assistance to save us.

There are labs to test your blood sugar, but things you experience every single day can also show you if your blood sugar needs some extra attention. Do you check off any of these boxes?

SIGNS OF BLOOD SUGAR DYSREGULATION

- Extreme thirst or hunger
- Urinating frequently
- Feeling weak or tired between meals
- Weight gain, inability to lose weight, or unintentional weight loss
- Acne or cystic acne

- Feeling hungry often, or shortly after a meal
- Consistent sugar cravings
- Hair thinning or hair loss
- Low libido
- Not having a daily bowel movement
- Waking up throughout the night
- Desire to overeat or binge on foods

- Dark, velvety skin on neck, armpits, or groin
- Blurred vision
- Feeling irritable or anxious
- Dizziness and sweating
- Shakiness if going too long between meals
- Heart palpitations

If you checked off at least three boxes, there's a good chance your blood sugar levels need extra attention.

To get even more information on your blood glucose levels, you can order labs, including:

Fasting glucose: This test measures the level of glucose (sugar) in your blood at that specific time. It can be measured with a finger prick or blood draw. Current medical guidelines recommend a level under 100 mg/dL, and the optimal range is between 72–85 mg/dL.

Fasting insulin: This test measures the level of insulin in your blood at a specific time and can monitor insulin resistance. This test is not as common as a fasting glucose test due to insulin being overlooked in our modern healthcare system. Because of that, there is not a scientific consensus on what an ideal number for fasting insulin should be. Some experts recommend a level under 10 µU/mL, while others recommend a value closer to 2–6 µU/mL.

Hemoglobin A1C: This test looks at the amount of sugar attached to a protein called hemoglobin for three consecutive months. Although everyone has some amount of sugar attached to hemoglobin, those with consistently higher blood sugar levels have a higher hemoglobin A1C value. This is a great test to assess overall blood sugar levels for a longer duration of time, and it is a common test used to diagnose prediabetes and type 2 diabetes. The following chart shows what the values mean.

Diagnosis	Hemoglobin A1C Level
Normal range	Below 5.7%
Prediabetes	5.7%–6.4%
Diabetes	6.5% and above

Source: National Institute of Diabetes and Digestive and Kidney Diseases 2018

I'd recommend getting these lab values checked at least annually to measure blood sugar status.

Another helpful way to look at your blood sugar levels is through a continuous glucose monitor (CGM). This allows you to look at your blood glucose levels at any time, or over a few hours or days. The CGM reviews your glucose level every couple of minutes and keeps track of it over time through a tiny sensor inserted under your skin (often on the arm or belly) or with an implantable sensor. This is a great way to see how certain foods impact your blood sugar and whether or not you're experiencing quick spikes or drops in your blood sugar throughout the day. Keep in mind that food is meant to raise blood sugar levels to a certain extent. What's most important is looking at the curve of your blood sugar levels during the day. Does it look like it has really high spikes and quick drops? Or does it look more like rolling hills? Ideally there should be no more than a 30 mg/dL increase from pre-meal levels. Foods impact everyone differently, and when I wore a CGM for two weeks, I learned a lot about how different foods impact my blood sugar levels throughout the day.

Continuous glucose monitors are typically only prescribed for those already diagnosed with prediabetes or diabetes, although they're available from private companies for those who desire to use it for preventable health.

WHAT IF YOUR BLOOD WORK IS NORMAL?

If it is, awesome! As I've mentioned before, even if your blood sugar labs come back as normal, I'd still focus on supporting your blood sugar levels for preventative health. Although lab work can be a really helpful tool, sometimes just tuning in to your own symptoms, like sugar cravings or your energy between meals, can be a powerful tool as well.

Oftentimes, it's easy to disregard common struggles as "normal" (like sugar cravings) just because they're common, when in fact, those struggles aren't always "normal." Moral of the story: lab testing can be a great tool, but it's important to pay attention to how you feel during the day as well.

Alright, so now that you know some signs that your blood sugar needs support, let's dive into HOW to begin optimizing your blood sugar with nutrition.

Quick tip: Lab tests can give great insight on blood sugar levels, but so can symptoms like energy levels, sugar cravings, sleep quality, hunger, and mood. Use the acronym SCHMEC (sleep, cravings, hunger, mood, energy, consistency) to assess yours on a daily basis.

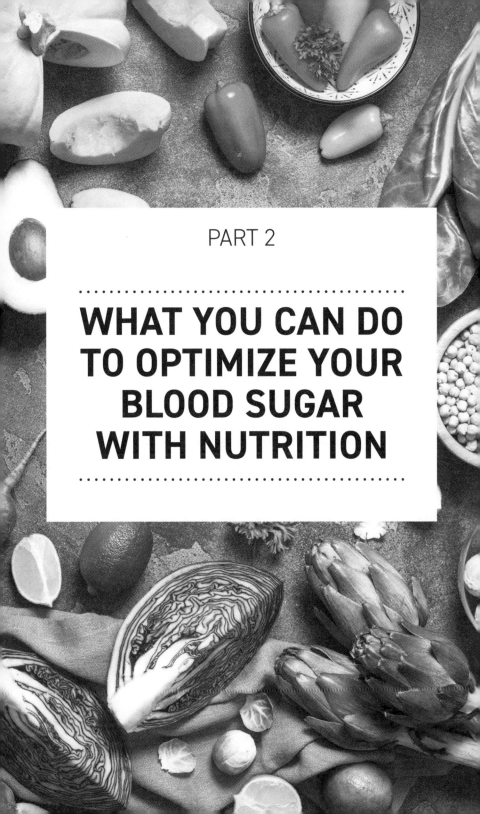

PART 2

WHAT YOU CAN DO TO OPTIMIZE YOUR BLOOD SUGAR WITH NUTRITION

CHAPTER 4

• • • • • • • • • • •

GETTING OFF THE BLOOD SUGAR ROLLER COASTER

"Inspiration exists, but it has to find you working."

—Pablo Picasso

"I'm anxious all the time, always feel like I need a sugar fix, and constantly want to eat." These are words I commonly hear from clients, and for my client Taylor, it was what she was struggling with every single day.

When Taylor first came to me, she was drinking a large vanilla latte for her breakfast. She wasn't really eating lunch either, but rather snacking here and there during the day. On top of that, she constantly felt stressed, overwhelmed, and anxious about everything. She was a busy working mom struggling to balance taking care of the kids and also taking care of her health.

If you can relate to that, know you aren't alone.

We're a society more stressed out than ever. We have way more things on our never-ending to-do list and constant pressures of making everything in our lives look nice and shiny. On top of that, our environment is set up to keep us even more unhealthy. With fast-food restaurants and convenience stores nearly on every corner, sitting at a desk all day as the "norm," and pills often prescribed over diet changes, no wonder we're exhausted, cranky, and just want to lie on the couch all night with a box of cookies.

The obesity rates have tripled over the past sixty years, with nearly 80 percent the US adult population either overweight or obese (USA Facts 2023). It's also estimated that roughly 60 percent of US adults have a chronic disease such as type 2 diabetes, cancer, heart disease, COPD, or irritable bowel syndrome (Centers for Disease Control and Prevention 2022). About five years ago, only 6.8 percent of the US population was found to be metabolically healthy, which is defined by "the absence of any metabolic disorder and cardiovascular disease, including type 2 diabetes, dyslipidemia, hypertension, and atherosclerotic cardiovascular diseases in a person with obesity" (Blüher 2020). This percentage will likely continue to decline with more individuals becoming increasingly sick.

These statistics are a representation of the need to take our health into our own hands. If our environment isn't set up to make living a healthy, vibrant lifestyle easy and accessible, then it's up to us to take over the wheel and be the drivers of our own health.

THE STANDARD AMERICAN DIET (SAD)

One of the first things I talked about with Taylor was the importance of balancing her blood sugar. The truth is, drinking a sugary coffee drink for breakfast, and the constant snacking all day, was fueling what I call the blood sugar roller coaster.

Sure, roller coasters are fun when you're little. There's the thrill and adrenaline rush of climbing up the railway slowly and then quickly dropping with sudden changes in speed and direction. My twelve-year-old self would have happily ridden it all day long. The problem is, many of us are experiencing that with our blood sugar every single day.

As I talked about in Chapter 1, every time you eat a carbohydrate, whether it's from a banana or donut, your body breaks down the carbohydrates into a type of sugar called glucose. Glucose then enters your bloodstream, which causes an increase in your blood sugar levels. At that time, your pancreas produces insulin, which helps the body use the glucose for energy or store it for later on. Now I'm not saying that bananas and donuts provide similar nutrient profiles, but it's important to know that all carbohydrates impact blood sugar in some way. Carbohydrates are your quick source of energy in your body, but finding the right balance and focusing on the right types of carbohydrates are key. So although the "fat will make you fat" trend has emerged into the "carbs are evil" era, I'm here to tell you, we do need to include carbohydrates during the day, but balance is key.

Most of the time carbohydrates are thought of as pastas, breads, donuts, and crackers, but carbohydrates are also found in vegetables, fruits, dairy, beans, and some nuts and seeds. With the Standard American Diet (aka SAD diet), though many people are not filling their bodies with these nourishing foods. It's estimated that 70–80 percent of calories consumed are in the form of carbohydrates; and I'm not talking about the colorful, nutrient-dense carbohydrates either. Think processed and convenience foods like chips, cookies, pasta dishes, crackers, and cereals. Think about it—you can hardly go anywhere without highly processed, sugary foods in site. Unfortunately, the chemicals, sugar, and additives in these foods negatively impact the body both internally and externally.

When the majority of the diet consists of carbohydrates, while lacking in high-quality proteins and nourishing fats, it's easy to ride on a blood sugar roller coaster all day. Just like any roller coaster, when it goes up the railway, it also has to come down. So what do you think happens when the day is started with a flavored coffee drink with fifty grams of sugar in it? Or if breakfast is consumed, what happens with foods like toast, waffles, or sugary granola bars? That roller coaster starts quickly going up that railway, and when it gets to the top, it drops quickly. Then when your blood sugar drops, it's like, *"Hey! I want more!"* and craves even more carbohydrates or sugar. The cycle then continues with constant highs and lows, snacking, and cravings.

It's no wonder when I used to follow the food pyramid *(remember those days?)* and start my day with whole grain cereal with skim milk, thinking it was a healthy choice, I was hungry an hour later. I would then snack on a banana *(again, another healthy choice, right?)* and be hungry shortly after that too. I was mainly fueling my body with carbohydrates without pairing it with any protein or nourishing fats to keep me feeling full. Carbohydrates by themselves will not keep you feeling full and satisfied, and that's what the majority of the Standard American Diet consists of.

So instead, if I would have taken that banana and mixed it with some plain Greek yogurt, guess what would have happened? I would have stayed full for a longer period of time, and my blood sugar wouldn't have gotten as big of a thrill ride compared to eating it alone.

Research has found this to be true as well. For example, one study compared glucose levels of individuals who ate just a carbohydrate alone to individuals who ate a carbohydrate paired with a protein source. Results found a significantly higher glucose level with the individuals who ate the carbohydrate alone without a protein source (Basturk et al. 2021). We'll talk more about balancing your meals and snacks in the next chapter, but one easy tip to support stable blood sugars is to *always pair your carbohydrate with a buddy.* Just as in grade school when we were always taught to "buddy up" in gym class, carbs also need a buddy. When you pair a protein or nourishing fat with the carbohydrate, it acts as a buffer to prevent such large spikes in your blood sugar. Better yet, it will keep you full for much longer and can help prevent cravings or snacking later on.

THE PROBLEM WITH DIETS

Now that you know the impact a diet high in carbohydrates (without a balance of protein or fat) can do to your blood sugar, let's talk about another common problem that can impact blood sugars . . . diets.

With weight loss being a 3.4 billion dollar industry, it's no shocker if you've ever been on a diet. In fact, over half (52 percent) of individuals between the ages of eighteen to thirty-four have tried a diet in the past year (IBIS World 2023). I remember going on my first diet at the age of eighteen, focusing on eating mainly cereal and cereal bars in an effort to lose weight for prom.

But here's the kicker: 95 percent of people who diet end up regaining all the weight (plus add on some additional weight) within two years of their diet. Why is that? Because the body is wired for survival, and not eating enough puts the body into a stressed state. Not only does this mean the body will slow down the metabolism in an effort to survive, it will also lead to increased hunger hormones (ghrelin) and decreased feelings of fullness (leptin). Remember those hormones? So not only are diets stressful for your metabolism, they also can influence your appetite hormones in a negative way.

Plus, low calorie consumption is stressful on your blood sugars. That's because if you don't eat enough for your body, it stays in a *hypoglycemic* state. Although this might sound like it would be beneficial for weight loss, having constant low blood sugars can trigger binging or overeating later on. Many people experience the diet-cycle hamster wheel:

They start a diet for a couple of weeks.

Then they get off the diet and binge on all the foods they missed while on the diet.

Then they feel guilty for binging and start another diet.

Then they continue the cycle of binging, guilt, and dieting.

Does that sound familiar?

Ultimately, what leads to the most effective and sustainable result is focusing on nourishing, wholesome foods while supporting your blood sugars with *how* you're eating.

Let's go back to my client Taylor. She wasn't eating anything for breakfast and was hardly eating a complete meal for lunch either. Instead, she was constantly having the urge to snack on food all day because she wasn't raising her blood sugar levels enough to feel full and satisfied. She needed to eat balanced and filling meals throughout the day to get to the point where her blood sugars were stable and she no longer had the desire to constantly snack.

And those sugar cravings? You can blame low blood sugar for that as well. That's because the body is really smart and is always trying to protect you. Remember how carbohydrates can raise your blood sugar? When your blood sugars are constantly in a low state, your body tends to crave more carb-heavy, sugary foods to raise it back up. Therefore, not eating enough calories for what your body needs leads to staying in a hypoglycemic state.

It's not ideal for the body to be in a *hyper* or *hypo*glycemic state. Instead, we want to find the right balance between the two.

Another common problem I see when it comes to blood sugars is following what I call the "weekday dieter" routine. The weekday dieter tends to "eat perfectly" during the week but gives in to anything and everything on the weekends. So their blood sugar is in a hypoglycemic state during the week and a hyperglycemic state on the weekends. Then Monday rolls around, and they are back to "starting over" in a low-calorie state. Instead, following strategies and methods to support stable blood sugars during the weekdays and weekends is going to be the most impactful for areas of weight loss, energy, hormone health, and reducing sugar cravings.

So, ready to dive in even further? Let's do it in the next chapter.

> **Quick tip:** Avoid eating carbohydrates alone to prevent blood sugar spikes and drops. Instead, pair carbohydrates with a protein or fat to feel full longer and maintain stable blood sugar levels.

CHAPTER 5
. . . .

BALANCING YOUR PLATE WITH PROTEIN, CARBOHYDRATES, AND FATS

"Let thy food be thy medicine and thy medicine be thy food."

—Hippocrates

Optimal blood sugars always begin with a balanced plate. We can balance our plate when we include all three macronutrients: protein, carbohydrates and fat. These macronutrients provide calories and unique functions that impact how you feel. They're all important in their own way, and the body is designed to have a balance of all three.

A SIMPLE METHOD TO BALANCING YOUR PLATE

As I mentioned in the last chapter, the Standard American Diet is rich in carbohydrates and lacks high-quality protein or fats. This can lead to large swings in blood sugar levels, causing increased hunger and calorie consumption. With popular diets like keto or low-fat diets, it's no wonder why most people are confused on what to even put on their plate. Although you can find studies showing the benefits of several ways of eating, whether it's low fat, low carb, or high protein, we don't need to go to the extreme by significantly reducing any of the macronutrients. We just need to learn how to balance our plates better, and we can do that with something called PFF.

PFF stands for protein, fat, and fibrous carbohydrates. When you can get your meals consisting of PFF, you'll be able to support stable blood sugar levels for a longer period of time. I hear from clients all the time that just this simple change has improved their energy, kept them feeling full longer, and reduced sugar cravings in a short amount of time.

WHY WE NEED A BALANCE OF ALL THREE MACRONUTRIENTS

Each macronutrient is important in its own unique way. Feeling hungry an hour after eating a meal? You may need to bump up your protein. Is your skin dry, or are you struggling with brain fog? You may need more fat. Feeling shaky or craving sugar all day? You may need more carbohydrates. When you have a balance of all three macronutrients, your blood sugars become balanced, and that, my friend, is where the sweet spot is.

So let's dive into each macronutrient, why it's important, and sources of each one.

PROTEIN

Protein is the macronutrient that most people don't consume enough of. I'm not saying we need to start eating protein like we're prepping for a bodybuilding competition, but many people are missing the benefits of protein simply by not having enough of it during the day.

BENEFITS OF PROTEIN

- Protein is a building block for every cell in the body and acts as a messenger for hormones.
- It helps decrease fat mass while preserving fat-free mass.
- It supports feeling full by reducing the hunger hormone *ghrelin*. Many of my clients tell me they feel less hunger after increasing their protein intake.

- Protein is also supportive of weight loss because of its higher thermic effect. This means that protein burns more energy (20–30 percent) compared to carbohydrates (5–10 percent) or fats (0–3 percent).
- It's also essential for a healthy immune system, reproduction, and muscle growth. That's because protein contains amino acids, which help promote muscle growth while preventing the loss of muscle mass.

Other notable differences protein can have include less sugar cravings; stronger hair, skin, and nails; more energy; and better mental focus.

HOW MUCH PROTEIN SHOULD YOU HAVE?

A great place to start with protein is to consume a serving size as large as the palm of your hand and the thickness of a deck of cards at each meal (or about twenty to thirty grams of protein per meal). For snacks, aim for about half that amount. Your protein needs change, depending on your health goals, age, sex, stress levels, activity, etc., but this is a great place to start. If that seems like a lot at first, start out slowly and work your way up to that amount.

SOURCES OF PROTEIN

- Meat and seafood—beef, poultry, pork, turkey, fish, shellfish
- Dairy products—milk, yogurt, cottage cheese, kefir, cheese
- Nitrate-free deli meats or jerky
- Eggs
- Nuts and seeds—peanuts, almonds, pistachios, sunflower seeds
- Nut butters—natural peanut butter, almond butter, or sunbutter
- Legumes—beans, lentils, peas
- Protein and collagen powders

Overall, animal sources will give you the most bang for your buck when it comes to the amount of protein per gram. If you're not into eating animals, know that sources like beans and lentils do provide protein, but they're also higher in carbohydrates. For example, one cup of cooked lentils provides almost eighteen grams of protein, but it also has about forty grams of carbohydrates. So if you're focusing on more plant-based proteins, it can be more challenging to get all your protein needs in.

When it comes to protein, the most important thing is to focus on *quality*. What you might see when you look at a grass-fed burger is just . . . a burger, although that grass-fed burger also contains nutrients like B vitamins, omega-3 fatty acids, zinc, iron, potassium, vitamin A, and more. Similarly, pasture-raised eggs with rich orange yolks contain higher amounts of vitamin A, E, and carotenoids (an antioxidant) compared to those in caged hens (Sergin 2022). The healthier the animal, the healthier the product is for us (we are literally what we eat).

I'm not saying all protein sources have to be grass-fed or organic. If your budget allows for it, great. If not, focus on lean varieties of meat (lean is better since toxins are stored in the fat cells), and focus on making simple switches. For example, try natural peanut butter made of just peanuts and salt instead of traditional peanut butter packed with oils and sugar, or tuna packed in water instead of oils, or plain Greek yogurt instead of regular flavored yogurts. These small changes can make a big difference.

HOW TO INCORPORATE MORE PROTEIN IN YOUR MEALS OR SNACKS

Since protein is typically the macronutrient that requires the most planning, I recommend planning your meals around your protein source first. Then you can balance your plate with carbohydrates and fat afterward.

Here are some examples:

○ Swap cereal or toast in the morning for an egg bake.

○ Add protein powder to oatmeal or a smoothie.

○ Switch from regular yogurt to Greek yogurt (it typically has more protein).

○ Add collagen powder to your morning coffee or tea.

○ Top salads with chicken or canned tuna.

○ Pair fruit with natural peanut butter or cheese for snacks.

Along with that, eating your protein first at a meal before any carbohydrates can help lower your spikes in blood sugar. That's because protein acts as a buffer and keeps blood glucose levels more stable. An example would be eating eggs first at breakfast before having toast or fruit.

CARBOHYDRATES

Although carbohydrates are often feared, the body needs carbohydrates—and the *type* of carbohydrate is what really matters. Carbohydrates come in the form of pastas and breads but also vegetables, fruit, and some dairy. Even certain nuts contain carbohydrates. If you're like me and dipped your toes in the low-carbohydrate scene while replacing all your rice with cauliflower rice and wraps with lettuce wraps, it may seem weird to be focusing on carbohydrates. They provide so many health benefits though.

BENEFITS OF CARBOHYDRATES

○ Carbohydrates provide a quick energy source for your body by breaking down into *glucose*—your body's main (and preferred) energy source.

○ They help control blood glucose and insulin metabolism, along with assisting in cholesterol and triglyceride metabolism.

○ Carbohydrates promote a healthy gut environment by fueling gut bacteria.

○ They support thyroid health because glucose is the main energy source for the pituitary gland and hypothalamus, which are the parts of your brain that regulate thyroid hormones.

○ Certain carbohydrates (like veggies and fruit) provide a source of fiber beneficial for reducing blood sugar levels, supporting satiety, and promoting heart health.

○ They support regulation of sex hormones, which play a key role in fertility, moods, and libido.

○ Carbohydrates help conserve muscle mass because carbohydrates are partially converted to glycogen, a form of energy stored in the muscles.

As you can see, carbohydrates play several key functions in the body. Carbohydrates come in all different forms, and focusing on the *type* is what matters the most.

THE DIFFERENT TYPES OF CARBOHYDRATES

SIMPLE CARBOHYDRATES

This type of carbohydrate is made with a shorter chemical structure and is quick to digest in the body, thus causing a rapid rise in blood sugar.

Common foods and beverages made with simple carbohydrates:

- Candy
- Sugary beverages such as soda, energy drinks, or ones made with fruit juice concentrate
- Syrups such as corn syrup or high fructose corn syrup
- Table sugar
- Cereals with added sugar
- Products made with refined flour
- Baked goods such as donuts or cookies

COMPLEX CARBOHYDRATES

This type is made with a longer chemical structure, which means they take longer for the body to break down. This type provides longer-lasting energy and helps prevent large spikes in blood sugar.

Common foods and beverages made with complex carbohydrates:

- Non-starchy vegetables such as broccoli, kale, green beans, or zucchini
- Starchy vegetables such as beets, carrots, sweet potatoes, or squashes
- Whole grains such as oats, quinoa, or brown rice
- Fruits such as apples, oranges, berries, and bananas
- Beans and lentils such as chickpeas, black beans, or kidney beans

As you can see, complex carbohydrates differ from simple carbohydrates because they contain more fiber and don't digest in the body as quickly. In other words, it slows down the absorption of carbohydrates and reduces the release of sugar in the body. This is ideal for blood sugar because it won't create those huge spikes and dips in glucose levels. When it comes to carbohydrates, focus on fiber-rich sources.

Currently, the average American only consumes about fifteen grams of fiber each day, but ideally we should be having more like twenty-five to thirty grams each day. Below is a table with fifteen sources of fiber.

Item	Serving Size	Fiber Amount (in grams)
Black beans (cooked)	1 cup	15
Green lentils (cooked)	1 cup	15
Chia seeds	2 tablespoons	10
Avocado	1 medium	10
Green peas	1 cup	9
Blackberries	1 cup	8
Pears	1 medium	6
Raspberries	1 cup	5
Broccoli	1 cup	5
Quinoa, cooked	1 cup	5
Apple	1 medium	4
Oatmeal	1 cup	4
Flaxseed	1 tablespoon	4
Almonds	¼ cup	4
Carrots	1 cup, sliced	3.5

Here's an example of how you could get at least twenty-five grams of fiber in a day:

- Add 1 tablespoon of chia seeds to a smoothie or yogurt (5 grams of fiber) with 1 cup blackberries (8 grams)
- Top a salad with ½ medium avocado (5 grams)
- Have 1 cup of broccoli at dinner (5 grams)
- Have ¼ cup almonds with a snack (4 grams)

Total fiber intake = 27 grams

HOW MANY CARBOHYDRATES DO YOU NEED?

I wish I could give you an exact number for how many carbohydrates you should have each day, but the truth is, everyone is so different. For example, a physically active individual would need more carbohydrates than someone not as active, or someone who is pregnant needs more carbohydrates than someone who isn't pregnant. Overall, your activity level, age, stress level, body size, sleep patterns, and genetics all play a role in the amount of carbohydrates you should have each day.

Generally speaking, someone following a well-rounded diet should consume about 30–40 percent of their diet from carbohydrates. Some may need more, and some may need less.

Your carbohydrate consumption can also fluctuate depending on the day. For example, if you go to a workout class, your body would benefit from more carbohydrates that day, compared to a less active day. Or if you're under a lot of stress, your body may crave more carbohydrates to help stimulate the production of the feel-good brain chemical called serotonin.

As mentioned in Chapter 4, aim to always pair your carbohydrate with a buddy (aka a protein or fat). This will not only keep you feeling full longer, but it will also prevent a large spike in your blood sugar. This could mean adding protein powder to your morning oatmeal or dipping your apple slices in some natural peanut butter for a snack.

FATS

I had a client once who was terrified of fats. Like many of us, she grew up in the "fat makes us fat" scene and felt like if she ate anything with fat it would go straight to her hips. We've been brainwashed to think that eating fat will make us fat, but that's not entirely true. The 1980s was a time when low-fat diets began to skyrocket in popularity, but looking at it now, we need to step back and ask ourselves, *"How did that really work out for us?"* Was fat the actual problem, or was it all the refined carbohydrates we were replacing the fat with?

Studies have found that a decline in the amount of fat consumed has corresponded with a massive *increase* in obesity. Dr. Water Willet, a professor at Harvard School of Public Health, said, "Diets high in fat do not appear to be the primary cause of the high prevalence of excess body fat in our society, and reductions in fat will not be a solution" (Willet and Leibel 2011).

Simply removing fat from our diets is not the solution because many low-fat diets are high in refined and sugary carbohydrates. As with carbohydrates, the *type* of fats is important to pay attention to, because not all fats are created equal.

Let's first dive into why not all fat is the enemy and all the health benefits that nourishing fats (from sources like extra-virgin olive oil or avocados) can provide us.

BENEFITS OF FATS

○ Fat helps the body absorb fat-soluble vitamins like vitamin A, D, and K, which means we need to eat fat to absorb these important vitamins.

○ They boost energy and help metabolize insulin more effectively.

○ They act as a building block for important hormones, including estrogen and testosterone.

○ Fat makes food more flavorful and keeps you feeling full longer since fat provides more energy per gram compared to carbohydrates or protein (fat contains nine calories per gram, whereas carbohydrates and protein contain four calories per gram).

- Fats support brain health since 60 percent of the brain is made of fat.
- They promote a healthy immune system by reducing stress and inflammation in the body.

THE DIFFERENT TYPES OF FAT

Fats come in various forms, and although I'm all about eating fat, it's important to know that not all fats will impact your body the same. There are some fats that are nourishing for your metabolism and blood sugar, and others that are harmful (especially trans fats). The World Health Organization found that trans fats increase the risk of death by 34 percent and coronary heart disease deaths by 28 percent. This is the most harmful type of fat, and it should be avoided completely (World Health Organization 2018). The following are fats recommended to focus on.

OMEGA-3 FATTY ACIDS

These are the queen of fats and should be the main fats in our diets. Omega-3s are called essential fatty acids because since the body cannot make them on their own, we must consume them through food. They provide a ton of health benefits, including protection against cardiovascular disease, certain cancers, Alzheimer's disease, age-related macular degeneration, rheumatoid arthritis, and attention-deficit/hyperactivity disorder. They also play a key role in hormone health, mental health, and immunity (National Institutes of Health 2022).

You can find omega-3 fatty acids in:

- Wild-caught fatty fish such as salmon, herring, tuna, mackerel, and sardines
- Some nuts and seeds, including hemp seeds, chia seeds, and walnuts
- Flaxseeds and flax oil
- Cod liver oil
- Meats and dairy products from grass-fed sources
- Pasture-raised eggs

MONOUNSATURATED FATS

These are another beneficial fat that aid in the protection against heart disease, certain cancers like breast cancer, and improving insulin sensitivity

(Seungyoun et al. 2016). A study looking at the difference between a high monounsaturated diet compared to a high carbohydrate diet found that those on the high monounsaturated diet had better glycemic control, blood pressure, and improved triglyceride levels and weight (Qian et al. 2016).

Monounsaturated fats are found in:

○ Avocados

○ Extra-virgin olive oil

○ Nuts such as almonds, hazelnuts, and pecans

○ Olives

○ Seeds including sesame and pumpkin

SOME SATURATED FATS

A common misconception about fat is that all saturated fat increases the risk for heart disease. Research has found that's not necessarily true.

A meta-analysis study of twenty-one different research articles found no significant evidence of dietary saturated fat to increase the risk of coronary heart disease or cardiovascular disease. As with anything, it's important to focus on the quality and amount of the saturated fat you have (Siri-Tarino et al. 2010).

Common sources of saturated fat include coconut oil, palm oil, butter, lard, cured and fatty meats, cheese, whole-fat dairy, pastries, and biscuits. Some of those saturated fats are beneficial, and some aren't so much. For example, coconut oil contains saturated fat, but it's also composed of about 65 percent medium chain triglycerides (MCT), a type of healthy fat that is quickly absorbed into the bloodstream and burned as fuel for the body. Studies have found that consuming MCTs may help reduce body fat and triglyceride levels (Xue et al. 2009). Additionally, coconut oil contains vitamin E and lauric acid, a component in breast milk that contains anti-microbial and antiviral properties. So would I recommend skipping out on these amazing benefits of coconut oil because it contains saturated fat? Of course not.

Overall, a diet high in saturated fats from fried foods, cured meats, fast food, and sugary baked goods is going to impact your health very differently compared to one rich in beneficial saturated fats from coconut oil or grass-fed meat. Now, I'm not saying to pull a Julia Child and add "more butter" to everything, but there's no need to cut out saturated fat from your diet completely.

Now, let's answer another common question you might be wondering: *"What about cholesterol?"* Saturated fats are often believed to raise cholesterol levels, so let's dive into this. First, cholesterol is a waxy substance that helps your body make cell membranes, hormones, and vitamin D. It also plays a key role in your brain health, including mood regulation, learning, and memory. Your body *needs* cholesterol, and low cholesterol levels can actually be harmful for your health. A main concern for cholesterol is that it was believed to increase the risk for cardiovascular disease. For years, we were told to decrease cholesterol in foods as much as possible. We were told that foods like eggs would increase cholesterol levels if we ate them. Extensive research has not shown evidence to support this claim though. The 2015–2020 Dietary Guidelines for Americans even removed the dietary cholesterol restriction of 300 milligrams per day due to the lack of evidence (Ghada 2018).

FATS TO DITCH

Now that you know not all fats are created equal, it's time to talk about the ones that *should* be avoided, and that includes refined vegetable oils along with trans fats (also known as partially hydrogenated or hydrogenated oils).

TRANS FATS

The Food and Drug Administration banned trans fats in products after finally confirming that they were not safe for human consumption. Why are trans fats not safe? For one, they destroy cell membranes and can increase the risk for coronary artery disease. They also negatively impact the brain and nervous system, specifically with how neurons in the body communicate with one another *(which is kind of a big deal)*. They can also diminish mental health and increase the risk for depression, cognitive decline, and even Alzheimer's disease (Ginter and Simko 2016).

Now, if you grew up on Hostess Cupcakes and microwave popcorn like I did, know that these are prime sources of trans fats. You can also still find trans fats in foods like frozen pizzas, vegetable shortenings and some margarines, certain coffee creamers, baked goods like biscuits or frozen pies, and ready-to-use frostings.

It's also important to know that the front of a food package doesn't always give you the whole picture. A food company can say "No trans fats!" on the front of the label, when in fact, the product still has trans fats. That's because as long as it has less than 0.5 grams of trans fat per serving, the company can say it has "zero grams of trans fats" on the product. Pretty misleading, if I say so myself. That's why it's important to read the ingredient list on the back of the package and look for words such as *partially hydrogenated* or *hydrogenated oils* (FDA 2003).

REFINED VEGETABLE OILS

These oils were introduced as a "healthier" alternative to fats like butter, but that's not the case. That's because vegetable oils are high in omega-6 fatty acids. Our body needs both omega-3 and omega-6 fatty acids, but the Standard American Diet gets plenty of omega-6 already—in fact, too much. About one hundred years ago, the ratio of omega-6 to omega-3 was around four to one. Presently, it's around twenty to one, with a much higher consumption of omega-6 than omega-3. Why is this not great? Because a higher amount of omega-6 creates more stress and inflammation in the body and can lead to a higher risk of allergies and autoimmune reactions (DiNicolantonio and O'Keefe 2021).

Another thing to consider with vegetable oils is how they're made. Take canola oil, for example. To make canola oil, a solvent called *hexane* is used to chemically extract the oil from the seeds. Hexane has been shown to be a neurotoxin in rats. Not sure if I want to pour dressing made with that on my salad.

Refined vegetables to avoid:
- Corn oil
- Soybean oil
- Canola oil
- Vegetable oil

- Cottonseed oil
- Safflower oil
- Sunflower oil

Fats to focus on (*indicates best oils for cooking):

- Extra-virgin olive oil*
- Avocado oil*
- Cold-pressed, unrefined coconut oil*
- High-oleic sunflower oil
- MCT oil
- Macadamia nut oil
- Grass-fed ghee*
- Grass-fed butter*
- Cod liver oil
- Flaxseed oil
- Nuts like plain walnuts, brazil nuts, cashews, pistachios, and almonds
- Seeds like plain sunflower, pumpkin, flaxseed, hemp, or chia seeds
- Natural nut butters
- Olives
- Avocados
- Coconut milk (from a can)
- Coconut butter
- Meats and dairy products from grass-fed sources
- Wild-caught fatty fish such as salmon, herring, tuna, mackerel, and sardines
- Pasture-raised eggs

HOW MUCH FAT DO YOU NEED?

A good rule of thumb for fat is to aim for one to two tablespoons at each meal. For example, add a tablespoon of ground flaxseed to your morning smoothie or add two tablespoons of chopped walnuts to Greek yogurt. Generally speaking, someone following a well-rounded diet should consume about 30 percent of their diet from nourishing fats. Some may need more, and some may need less. Fats do contain more calories per gram compared to carbohydrates or protein, and they can add up quickly, so be mindful about overall intake.

Some signs you need more fat in your diet include dry, itchy skin, brain fog, difficulty focusing, constant fatigue, feeling cold often, achy and stiff joints, or brittle nails and hair. Along with that, lab values like low high-density lipoprotein (HDL) levels are a sign to bump up your consumption of beneficial fats. Some signs you need to cut back on fats include oily, floating stools, if you have problems with your gallbladder or have had it removed, or if you've had a stool test indicating fat malabsorption.

PUTTING IT ALL TOGETHER: CREATING A PFF-BALANCED MEAL

Now that we've gone through all the macronutrients, the benefits of each one, and sources of them, let's put them all together with a PFF-balanced meal.

For optimal blood sugar support, aim to make your meals:

- Half fibrous, non-starchy vegetables (such as broccoli, green beans, or salad)
- One-fourth high-quality protein (or about a palm-size amount)
- One-fourth starchy carbohydrate (such as fruit, rice, potatoes, pasta, or squashes)
- One to two tablespoons of nourishing fat (like avocado slices, nuts, seeds, or cooking oil)

Below is an example of what a blood-sugar friendly, balanced PFF meal could look like:

PFF-BALANCED PLATE

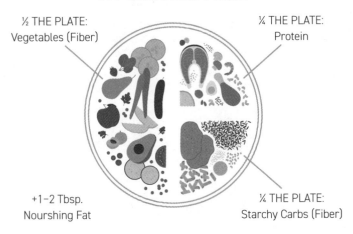

½ THE PLATE:
Vegetables (Fiber)

¼ THE PLATE:
Protein

+1–2 Tbsp.
Nourishing Fat

¼ THE PLATE:
Starchy Carbs (Fiber)

Not every meal may look exactly like this, and that's okay. Just focus on getting the basics down with protein, fibrous carbohydrates, and nourishing fats.

WHAT ABOUT SNACKS?

Snacks can get a bad reputation, but they can actually help optimize your blood sugar if you're using them correctly. It can be helpful to add in a snack between meals if your meals are spaced out over five or six hours apart. For example, if you eat breakfast at seven a.m. and don't have lunch until one p.m., it may be helpful to add a mid-morning snack around ten a.m. to keep blood sugars stable, and to not go too long without eating. That's because if we go too long without eating, blood sugar levels drop. Your body then starts to crave sugar or carbs to help raise it back up. This can lead to overeating or binging on food later on—a common struggle I hear from clients who skip meals or don't have time to eat. Snacks are often thought of as foods like chips or crackers, but it's best to focus on snacks that will sustain our energy and support stable blood sugars. When it comes to snacks, focus on fiber-rich carbohydrates (like a vegetable or fruit) with a protein. This is what I call PF.

Here are some examples of how to do that:

○ Greek yogurt with blueberries

○ One hard-boiled egg with carrots

○ One apple with almond butter mixed with hemp seeds

○ Cucumbers with tuna

Snacks can be helpful for supporting stable blood sugars, but keep in mind, snacking all day long (aka grazing) is not beneficial for blood sugar or your health, for that matter. We need to give the body time to rest and digest, and if we're constantly snacking, it's hard for the body to do that. So, remember to allow a couple of hours between your meals and snacks to let your body have a break.

WHAT WOULD THIS LOOK LIKE IN REAL LIFE?

Here are some examples of what balanced meals and snacks could look like.

○ **Breakfast:** a piece of egg bake made with eggs, spinach, and broccoli. Serve with a side of sourdough toast and avocado

- **Mid-afternoon snack:** cottage cheese with a pear
- **Lunch:** salad with grilled chicken, broccoli, carrots, tomatoes, and sunflower seeds. Serve with an olive-oil based dressing and an apple on the side
- **Mid-afternoon snack:** plain Greek yogurt with blueberries, cinnamon, and a little raw honey
- **Dinner:** burrito bowl made with romaine lettuce, peppers, tomatoes, black beans, grass-fed hamburger, avocado, and salsa

Check out the recipes in the back of the book for more PFF-balanced meals and snacks, and get a free downloadable macronutrient guide at https://autumnenloe.com/bloodsugarbook.

> **Quick tip:** Focus on having a protein, fat, and fibrous carbohydrate (PFF) at meals, and a protein with a fibrous carbohydrate at snacks (PF).

REFLECTION

1. What do your current meals and snacks typically look like? Write them below. Could they be more balanced? If so, how?

CHAPTER 6

THE GLYCEMIC INDEX OF FOODS

"When we strive to become better than we are, every-thing around us becomes better too."

—Paulo Coelho

In the carbohydrate section in the previous chapter, I talked about the difference between simple and complex carbohydrates. Now we're going to take it a step further and dig deeper into how carbohydrates impact your blood sugars, using the glycemic index.

UNDERSTANDING THE GLYCEMIC INDEX

The glycemic index of foods (often shortened to "GI") is a scaling system, between one and one hundred, used to represent how high blood glucose levels rise two hours after consuming food. Consuming foods with a high glycemic index can cause blood glucose and insulin levels to spike quickly, whereas foods listed with a low glycemic index

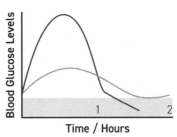

Time / Hours

Source: Harvard Medical School 2012, www.health. harvard.edu/healthbeat/a-good-guide-to-good -carbs-the-glycemic-index

number (fifty-five and under) don't cause as large a spike. The image on the right is an example.

To determine the GI of food, participants are given a test food and control food (such as pure glucose) on separate dates. Both the test food and control food contain fifty grams of carbohydrates. Changes in blood glucose and insulin are then measured every two hours, and the GI of the test food is then calculated. The glycemic index captures the impact certain foods have on blood sugar and insulin levels. Over the past three decades, several thousand food items have been measured on the glycemic index scale (Harvard Medical School 2012).

Although the impact on carbohydrates can differ with each individual, as well as what other food and drink the carbohydrate is served with, the concept of the glycemic index can be a helpful tool when selecting the best carbohydrates to support your blood sugar balance. For example, a serving of white rice will spike your blood sugar higher than a serving of lentils due to the lack of fiber the white rice contains.

Researchers have found other benefits to using the glycemic index as well. For example, a study looking at over 137,000 participants found that those who ate foods with a high glycemic index had an increased risk for cardio-vascular disease and mortality (Jenkins et al. 2021). Other studies have found low-GI eating patterns to be helpful at reducing hemoglobin A1C values, fasting glucose, body mass index (BMI), total cholesterol, and LDL (Zafar et al. 2019).

Some countries like Australia and New Zealand have even adopted the concept of the glycemic index on their food packaging with a symbol to inform consumers whether it's a low-GI food. Imagine how shopping habits would change if consumers knew the impact certain foods would have on their blood sugars versus just relying on things like calories or terms like "heart healthy" (Barclay et al. 2021).

Plus, it's easy. If you are someone who likes to have lists, using the glyce-mic index can be a great, simple tool for you.

EXAMPLES OF FOODS IN EACH CATEGORY

LOW GLYCEMIC INDEX (55 AND UNDER)

- Fruits like apples, avocados, oranges, berries, peaches, pears, and plums
- Vegetables such as broccoli, cauliflower, zucchini, peppers, spinach, carrots, lettuce, butternut squash, yams, parsnips, and artichokes
- Beans, including black, kidney, pinto, and chickpeas, as well as lentils
- Grains like sourdough, whole grain tortillas, quinoa, steel-cut oats, and popcorn
- Dairy, including cottage cheese, plain greek yogurt, cow's milk, and non-dairy milk (like almond milk)
- Nuts and seeds such as almonds, peanuts, cashews, pistachios, pumpkin seeds, sunflower seeds, chia seeds, and flaxseed
- Sweeteners like dates, maple syrup, manuka honey, and coconut sugar

MODERATE GLYCEMIC INDEX (56 TO 69)

- Fruits like ripe bananas, cherries, mangoes, grapes, kiwi, and pineapples
- Vegetables such sweet potatoes, pumpkins, potatoes, and beets
- Grains like brown, basmati, and wild rice, quinoa, farro, muesli, instant oats, and cornmeal, as well as breads like pumpernickel, rye, and pita bread

HIGH GLYCEMIC INDEX (70 AND HIGHER)

- Fruits like watermelon and overripe bananas
- Grains like white rice, whole wheat or white bread, cereal, bagels, rice cakes, crackers, and desserts like cakes or donuts
- Non-dairy milks like oat milk and rice milk
- Sweeteners like cane sugar

Get a free printable glycemic index guide at https://autumnenloe.com /bloodsugarbook.

SHOULD YOU ONLY EAT FOODS WITH A LOW GLYCEMIC INDEX VALUE?

While this book is focused on helping you improve your blood sugar, I'm also realistic. If you can aim for the majority of your carbohydrates to come from the low glycemic index category, that's great. If you enjoy one in the high glycemic index category (like my favorite, an oat milk latte) once in a while, that's okay too.

I would suggest avoiding eating foods with a high GI in the morning and before bed. That's because if you start your morning with a high GI food like cereal, for example, it's going to cause a blood sugar spike first thing in the morning. This can contribute to more blood sugar spikes and crashes later on. Before bed, I'd suggest focusing on low GI foods to help keep blood sugar stable throughout the night.

Also, when it comes to sweets like cookies or cakes, I'd suggest having them after a meal versus on an empty stomach. That way, the meal you consumed will help slow down the absorption of the sugar from the sweets. On the flipside, if you eat sweets on an empty stomach, you'll be riding that blood sugar roller coaster for a while.

WHO SHOULD USE THE GLYCEMIC INDEX?

Anyone! As you can see, there are plenty of carbohydrate options rated with a low GI value. This can be a great tool for those with blood sugar dysregulation, whether it's elevated glucose spikes or large dips in blood sugars. If you struggle with hypoglycemia, focusing on small, frequent meals and snacks and foods with a low GI value can also be helpful for stabilizing blood sugar levels.

Incorporating the glycemic index scale can not only help improve blood sugar levels, it can also be supportive for improving areas like energy, hormone health, digestion, weight, heart health, moods, and much more.

Quick tip: Aim to have the majority of your foods come from the low-to-moderate glycemic index categories.

CHAPTER 7

THE MAGIC OF VITAMINS AND MINERALS

"When health is absent, wisdom cannot reveal itself, art cannot manifest, strength cannot fight, wealth becomes useless, and intelligence cannot be applied."

—Herophilus

"I just can't lose weight no matter what I do." Melanie came to me after years of dieting and restricting calories in an effort to lose weight. She would lose weight for a short period of time but shortly gain it all back after she went to her old patterns. This is a common scenario. When calories are the main focus instead of quality of food, it's easy to lack essential vitamins and minerals in your diet. This lack of vitamins and minerals can increase the risk for developing chronic diseases, including heart disease, type 2 diabetes, osteoporosis, certain cancers, and depression. That's why a balance of macronutrients, with a variety of color and variation at your meals, is one of the best things you can do for your health (World Health Organization 2003).

I'm guessing you've heard of vitamins like vitamin C to help with immunity or vitamin D to help with mood. All the thirteen essential vitamins have different jobs to help keep your body strong and healthy. Some will fight off infection, while others will help boost your energy and fight off inflammation. There is no one "magic vitamin" that can do all the work. That's why it's essential to eat a variety of foods in order to obtain a variety of nutrients (National Institute of Aging 2021).

Minerals like potassium, magnesium, iron, phosphorus, and calcium are also critical for optimal health. Minerals are elements that are necessary for building bones, supporting muscle growth and nerve function, and regulating water balance in the body. They're also a key driver for hormones and supporting the body's immune system and blood sugar levels. Some minerals are needed more than others (like magnesium and potassium, for example), but obtaining a variety of foods to get an array of minerals is key (Weyh et al. 2022). Along with food, one way I personally love to get an extra dose of nourishing minerals is through "mineral mocktails." See the beverage recipes in the back (page 150) for ideas.

Let's dive into some of the most significant vitamins and minerals for blood sugars and how to obtain them in your diet.

VITAMINS

VITAMIN C

Although often thought of for its immune support, it does so much more than that. Not only is it required for metabolizing protein, it's also key for wound healing and reducing free radicals in the body with its antioxidant effect. The adrenal glands also need vitamin C to make hormones like cortisol and adrenaline. When it comes to supporting blood glucose levels, one study found that those who took vitamin C for twelve weeks improved hemoglobin A1C levels significantly (Dakhale et al. 2011).

Sources of vitamin C include:

- Bell peppers
- Oranges and 100 percent orange juice
- Kiwi
- Strawberries
- Broccoli
- Brussels sprouts

VITAMIN D

This fat-soluble vitamin (or sunshine vitamin) is also considered a hormone due to its role in many processes in the body. Vitamin D can be obtained from foods, supplements, and through the skin after exposure to ultraviolet B radiation. It plays an important role in the immune system, heart health, and hormones (Ellison and Moran 2021). It also helps with absorption of calcium, reducing inflammation, may help prevent cancer and slow tumor progression, and supports glucose metabolism. One of the most popular attributes of vitamin D is its role in mental health. Studies have found low levels of vitamin D to increase symptoms of depression and anxiety. If you live in a climate with gloomy, cold winters like I do, you may be familiar with the "winter blues." When we aren't getting consistent exposure to vitamin D, it can increase our risk for anxiety, depression, and, of course, motivation to get things done (Akpınar and Karadag 2022).

Along with sunlight, you can get vitamin D through foods like:

- Cod liver oil
- Trout, sardines, or salmon
- Mushrooms
- Dairy products
- Eggs

I recommend getting tested annually to monitor your vitamin D levels. An optimal range for vitamin D is between 50–80 ng/mL (National Institutes of Health 2023).

VITAMIN E

This is a fat-soluble vitamin and powerful antioxidant, meaning it helps reduce free radicals in the body. It also supports immunity, helps the body use vitamin K, and helps prevent blood clotting. It's also been found to reduce levels of hemoglobin A1C and fasting insulin in individuals with type 2 diabetes (Asbaghi et al. 2023, National Institutes of Health 2021).

You can find vitamin E in foods such as:

- Sunflower seeds
- Almonds
- Hazelnuts
- Peanuts

FOLATE

This is a water-soluble B vitamin, also known as folic acid (although this is a synthetic form). Your body needs folate to make DNA and other genetic material. It also plays a role in helping the body convert food into fuel (glucose) that can be used for energy (National Institutes of Health 2022).

A review of eighteen trials with over twenty-one thousand people with or without diabetes showed folate to be beneficial for decreasing fasting glucose levels and insulin resistance (Zhao et al. 2018).

Foods containing folate:
- Beef liver
- Broccoli
- Brussels sprouts
- Asparagus
- Leafy greens such as spinach, romaine lettuce, and turnip greens
- Peanuts
- Kidney beans

MINERALS

MAGNESIUM

My favorite mineral of them all is this one right here. Magnesium is one of the most abundant minerals in the body and plays a key role in everything from muscle health, blood pressure regulation, absorbing vitamin D in the body, energy production, and blood glucose control. It's a cofactor for over three hundred different processes in the body, and up to 50 percent of the American population is deficient in this important mineral. There are several different forms of magnesium, so the following is a breakdown of some of the most common types.

Common magnesium types:
- **Magnesium glycinate:** the most absorbable form of magnesium, this is great for supporting sleep, mood, and hormone health.
- **Magnesium citrate:** a common form of magnesium in products, this one is best for constipation since it's not absorbed as well and pulls water into the intestines.

○ **Magnesium chloride:** this is commonly found in lotions and topical sprays since it's well absorbed in the body.

○ **Magnesium malate:** another great absorbable form, this one is great for improving energy levels.

○ **Magnesium L-threonate:** this form can be helpful for brain health and memory.

○ **Magnesium taurate:** one of the best forms for blood sugar regulation, this form also supports heart health and healthy blood pressure.

○ **Magnesium sulfate:** this form is typically found in Epsom salts, and it is great for muscle soreness and relieving stress.

Along with supplemental magnesium, magnesium can be found in a variety of foods.

Foods containing magnesium:

○ Nuts like almonds, peanuts, and cashews

○ Seeds like pumpkin, sesame, and flaxseed

○ Black beans and kidney beans

○ Geens like spinach and swiss chard

○ Bananas

○ Brown rice

○ Oats

POTASSIUM

This is another essential mineral because it plays a role in nearly everything your body does, including regulating blood pressure, supporting bone health, muscle contraction, mental health, and insulin production in the pancreas. Low levels of potassium can negatively affect insulin secretion, and some studies have found lower levels of potassium to increase the risk for diabetes (Chatterjee et al. 2011).

Foods containing potassium:

○ Dried fruit like apricots and raisins

○ Root vegetables, including squash and potatoes

○ Leafy greens such as spinach and beet greens

○ Dairy products

○ Beans and lentils

○ Coconut water

ZINC

This mineral is naturally present in foods, added to others, and also available in supplement form. Often thought to enhance the immune system, it's also important for wound healing, DNA synthesis, taste, and healthy growth and development during pregnancy and beyond.

Zinc can also be supportive for blood sugar. For example, a review of fifteen studies found a positive effect on glycemic control with adequate zinc levels (Barbosa de Carvalho 2017). Other meta-analysis studies have found supplementing with zinc to be beneficial for reducing fasting blood glucose, hemoglobin A1C, triglycerides, total cholesterol, and LDL cholesterol levels (National Institutes of Health 2022).

Foods containing zinc:
- Shellfish like oysters, crab, and lobster
- Meats like beef, poultry, turkey, and pork
- Legumes
- Pumpkin seeds
- Cheddar cheese

CALCIUM

Another abundant mineral in the body, calcium plays a key role in bone health, helping your muscles move, supporting blood circulation, helping your nerves transmit messages throughout the body, and supporting hormone secretion.

Calcium works with vitamin D to optimize glucose metabolism, so getting a combination of both calcium and vitamin D is essential for blood sugar support (Pittas et al. 2007).

Foods containing calcium:
- Dairy such as milk, yogurt, cottage cheese, and cheese
- Canned sardines and salmon
- Almonds
- Greens such as spinach, turnip greens, bok choy, and kale
- Edamame
- Chia seeds
- Eggshell powder

Although cow's milk typically gets the credit for keeping bones strong, if you're sensitive to dairy, you can still obtain it through non-dairy sources.

GET A VARIETY OF NUTRIENTS WITH THE "3x3x3 METHOD"

Although all vitamins and minerals provide benefits, these are some of the most important when it comes to supporting blood sugar levels.

A tool I use with my clients to help bump up nutrients in their meals is what I call the "3x3x3 method"—eat all three macronutrients, with three different colors on your plate, three times per day. When you follow this simple method, it's easy to incorporate a variety of vitamins and minerals throughout your day.

REFLECTION

1. How can you add more of these vitamins and minerals into your meals and snacks? Write some ideas below.

Be sure to check out the recipe section starting on page 124 for help!

CHAPTER 8

WHAT ABOUT SUGAR?

"We are what we repeatedly eat. Healthy eating then, is not an act, but a habit."

—Felicity Luckey

"I feel like a total sugar addict, and I don't know how to stop!" My client Emily came to me with rising blood sugar levels, high blood pressure, and an intense sweet tooth. Her goal was to start losing weight in a healthy way without giving up all her favorite foods, lower her risk for diabetes, and get off her blood pressure medications. One of the first places she wanted to tackle was her sugar cravings.

If you can relate to Emily's story, ask yourself these questions:

○ Do you feel like you need a sugar fix each day?

○ Are you relying on sugar to give you the quick energy you need to get through your day (especially in the afternoon)?

○ Do you have a hard time understanding how someone can "just stop at one"?

○ Are you raiding your kitchen cabinet for the sweet stuff at night?

○ Do you crave sugar when you're feeling stressed, sad, or bored?

If you said "yes!" to any of the questions above, you're not alone. The average American consumes at least five to six tablespoons, or about 270 calories, each day from just sugar. This leads to over sixty pounds of sugar each year (Harvard 2022). Imagine pouring yourself a nice glass of sugar for breakfast. Not so nourishing is it? Yet many of the traditional breakfast meals are loaded with sugar. Not only does this trigger more sugar cravings later in the day, it also causes your blood sugars to go on a roller-coaster ride.

IT'S NOT ABOUT WILLPOWER

So often we tell ourselves we just "need more willpower," but anyone who has gone on a strict diet most likely has experienced a failure of willpower. Oftentimes we deny ourselves particular foods, and suddenly we can't take it any longer, and the floodgates open. Weekdays of salads and chicken result in weekends of pizza and take-out. Relying on willpower alone is exhausting and never the answer because it's so much more than that. Sugar can be addictive, and the more we consume it, the more we crave it. So it's not that you "just need more willpower" to stop eating it. What's most important is supporting your biochemistry, creating different habits around sugar, and nourishing your body well so you can stop craving sugar so much. Taste buds change every ten to fourteen days, so when you start changing your eating habits, your taste buds' preferences also change.

So now that you know that sugar cravings aren't because you're low on willpower, let's first dive into some actual culprits of sugar cravings.

Blood sugar imbalance: Not surprising to you at this point, I'm sure! This is one of the most common reasons for sugar cravings I see with clients. If your blood sugars are riding on high all day, sugar cravings tend to be like a clock tick-tocking in the background. On the flip side, if you don't eat enough calories, or enough macronutrients (like protein, for example), blood sugars tend to run low. When they dip too low, your body starts to crave sugar and carbohydrates to get it back up.

Lack of sleep: Sleep is an important time for the body to recharge. Without enough sleep, every system, organ, and hormone is impacted—including your appetite hormones. For example, ghrelin (your hunger hormone) becomes elevated when you don't get enough "zzzzz's" at night. That's often why you may feel more hungry or have more cravings the next day after a night of not-so-great sleep.

Nutrient deficiencies: Sometimes cravings can be a sign your body is trying to tell you something. For example, craving chocolate can signal your body needs more magnesium, or craving nut butters can be a sign that you're not eating enough fat. I also see a lack of protein intake during the day as a huge reason for sugar cravings.

Emotions: Sometimes we use sugar as a way to cope with emotions. Ever eat that brownie or cookie because you were feeling stressed or had a hard day at work? I definitely have. I'll dive more into this in the next chapter, but it can help to pause and consider if your sugar craving is a physical craving (your body actually needs more fuel or is low in something) or a head craving (you're eating out of emotion).

It's a habit: Sometimes we have cravings just because they've become a habit. For example, maybe you're used to always having a piece of chocolate after dinner, or used to grabbing a handful of candy from the candy dish after lunch. Sometimes these habits are just automatic without us even realizing it.

Consuming high amounts of sugar in foods and beverages: This is an obvious one, but I see many people eating and drinking foods and beverages with a lot of sugar and not even realizing it. For example, a small container of flavored yogurt can have as much as thirty grams of sugar, and a coffee drink can have as much as fifty grams of sugar. Even foods that may be considered "healthy" can actually be loaded with sugar. Granola, bars, salad dressings, and pre-made smoothies are some examples. All of these foods and beverages add up quickly.

It's not that you can never have sugar again (in fact, it's pretty impossible to avoid it completely), but starting to pay attention to sources of sugar in your foods and beverages is key. Let's first start with the nutrition facts label.

READ YOUR LABELS

Food marketing can be really convincing. Oftentimes, we just look at the front of a food package and believe the claims that are listed. I encourage you to find the real information on the back of the label though. Looking at the nutrition facts label and ingredient list on the back of the package will give you a lot more insight into the health of the product versus simply trusting what the front of the package says. During my dietetic internship I had a rotation with a major food company, and one of my tasks was to research what food companies are allowed to put on the front of their packages. Let's just say, the regulations are tricky and can be misleading.

For example, all the ingredients are listed in descending order of weight, with the first ingredient being used in the greatest amount, followed by those in smaller amounts (FDA 2023). So if a food company is using a lot of sugar in their product, they can make it look "healthier" by using several different forms of sugar in the product. That way, sugar won't be listed as one of the main ingredients in the product. Cane sugar is a common form of sugar, but there are also several names for sugar (fifty-six, in fact!).

Here are some examples:

○ Anything with "ose" at the end of it, such as sucrose, maltose, lactose, glucose, and fructose

○ Syrups like brown rice syrup, corn syrup, malt syrup, rice syrup, and high-fructose corn syrup

○ Juices like cane juice or fruit juice

○ Sugar from foods like coconut sugar, date sugar, or grape syrup

○ Artificial sweeteners like sucralose, aspartame, saccharine, neotame, and acesulfame potassium

Although I don't expect you to remember every single name for sugar, reviewing the ingredient list for words like "syrups" or words with "ose" is a great starting point. Another thing to pay attention to is the added sugar of the product. Some products naturally have sugar in them. For example, yogurt contains lactose, the type of sugar found in dairy products. A plain yogurt could have six to eight grams of natural sugar in it already. That's why I said earlier it's pretty impossible to eliminate sugar from your diet completely. What's important is to pay attention to what food companies are *adding* to the product. You can do this by simply looking right at the label.

Here's an example of a nutrition facts label. One of the most important sections to pay attention to for optimal blood sugars is the carbohydrate section. Carbohydrates are made of fiber, sugar, added sugar, and starches. In this example, you can see that there are a total of twelve grams of sugar, with ten of those grams being added. Naturally the product has two grams, and then the rest are being added to the product. Generally, I recommend trying to limit ten grams of added sugar per serving, and no more than twenty-five grams of total added sugar during the day.

Another important thing to mention is the serving size. In this example, one serving is two-thirds cup, and there are eight servings per container. So if you had two servings of this product, your total added sugar intake would go up from ten grams to twenty grams. *See how easily sugar can add up throughout the day?*

Nutrition Facts

8 servings per container

Serving size   **2/3 cup (55g)**

Amount per serving

Calories   **230**

	% Daily Value*
Total Fat 8g	**10%**
Saturated Fat 1g	**5%**
Trans Fat 0g	
Cholesterol 0mg	**0%**
Sodium 160mg	**7%**
Total Carbohydrate 37g	**13%**
Dietary Fiber 4g	**14%**
Total Sugars 12g	
Includes 10g Added Sugars	**20%**
Protein 3g	
Vitamin D 2mcg	10%
Calcium 260mg	20%
Iron 8mg	45%
Potassium 240mg	6%

* The % Daily Value (DV) tells you how much a nutrient in a serving of food contributes to a daily diet. 2,000 calories a day is used for general nutrition advice.

Source: FDA 2023

ARE THERE HEALTHIER OPTIONS FOR SUGAR?

This is a common question I get, and the answer is yes. I'm all about baking some banana bread or pumpkin muffins during the cooler months, and adding natural sugars can help enhance the flavor.

Here's an overview of how different sugars are rated on the glycemic index scale (which I talked about in Chapter 6):

Name of Sugar	Glycemic Index Value
Glucose	100
High-fructose corn syrup	87

Name of Sugar	Glycemic Index Value
Table sugar	80
Corn syrup	75
Brown sugar	70
Sucrose	65
Manuka honey	55
Maple syrup	54
Coconut sugar	50
Lactose	45
Xylitol	12
Stevia	>2
Monk fruit	0
Erythritol	0

As you can see, sugars will impact your glucose levels very differently. I personally love to use maple syrup, raw honey, or coconut sugar when I'm baking, despite the higher glycemic index value. When you combine these sweeteners with other ingredients like oats or flaxseed that contain fiber, they won't spike your blood sugar as much.

WHAT ABOUT STEVIA, ERYTHRITOL, OR MONK FRUIT?

Stevia is a sweetener naturally found on plants. There's a big difference between the stevia you can grow on a plant and the type of stevia you often find at the grocery store though. That's because many products labeled as "Stevia" at the grocery store are made from a highly refined stevia leaf extract called rebaudioside A (Reb-A) versus true stevia and also contain other ingredients like erythritol. Erythritol is considered an artificial sweetener that has been linked to increased risk of heart attack and stroke (National Institutes of Health 2023).

Monk fruit is a newer type of sweetener with a sugar-like consistency and light beige color. It can be one-hundred to two-hundred times sweeter than regular sugar, which can alter your taste buds to crave more sweet things. It can also be found mixed with other sweeteners like erythritol.

WHAT ABOUT ARTIFICIAL SWEETENERS?

When you're trying to cut down on your sugar consumption, artificial sweeteners like Splenda or aspartame may seem like the next "sweet" option. Unfortunately, they can be one of the worst things for you. You can find artificial sweeteners in products often labeled with terms like "sugar-free," "fat-free," "diet," "reduced sugar," or "zero sugar."

I commonly hear clients say they'll switch their regular soda for diet soda to be healthier and cut their sugar intake. Although they have the best intentions, making the switch to diet soda that contains artificial sweeteners can actually cause you to crave sugar even more. Some studies have even found diet soda to significantly increase the risk for developing diabetes (Fagherazzi et al. 2017).

Why would that be the case? That's because artificial sweeteners can be two hundred to six hundred times sweeter than regular sugar. Because of the intense sweetness, it's easier to crave more sugar. Remember how I said taste buds change every ten to fourteen days? When your taste buds get used to a really sweet taste, it's easy to crave it more.

Not only can artificial sweeteners cause *more* sugar cravings, they can also negatively impact your gut microbiome. Studies have found artificial sweeteners to change the composition and diversity of the gut microbiome, leading to decreased satiety, increased caloric intake, and altered glucose metabolism (Pearlman 2017, Nettleton et al. 2016). No thanks.

Let's not forget that the term "artificial sweetener" has *artificial* right in it. If you can remember only one thing from this book, remember that the body is designed to metabolize and digest real, wholesome foods—not food or food products made in a laboratory and designed to trick the body into wanting more.

> **Quick tip:** Aim for no more than ten grams of added sugar per serving, and no more than twenty-five grams of added sugar during the day.

REFLECTION

1. Think of some of the most common foods and beverages you consume. Now, take the next step and look at how much sugar they contain, if the information is available. For example, if you always get a morning latte at a coffee shop, look at the menu and see how much sugar is in it. Or if you always have flavored oatmeal or cereal in the morning, how much sugar is found in that?

2. Next, what are some ways you can reduce your total sugar intake each day? Maybe it's to swap your soda for carbonated water or to switch from flavored yogurt to plain yogurt and add your own flavoring (like a little maple syrup or berries). List some ways you can lower your sugar intake below.

CHAPTER 9

BREAKFAST AND BLOOD SUGARS

"But the real secret to lifelong good health is actually the opposite: Let your body take care of you."

—Deepak Chopra

Is breakfast *really* the most important meal of the day?

A common phrase I hear from clients is that they never feel hungry in the morning, so they skip breakfast each day. And with trends like intermittent fasting, skipping breakfast has become increasingly popular.

Here's the thing—your body has already been fasting overnight. Breakfast is called "breakfast" because it's there to literally *break the fast*. When you wake up, it's hard to expect the body to do things like prepare for your morning work meeting or stay calm despite all the chaos of getting the kids to school without fueling the tank first. Your body needs more than coffee for breakfast. Without proper fuel in the morning, you increase your chances of overeating later on, having more sugar cravings, fatigue, and having a hard time concentrating. Let's not forget the impact it can have on your blood sugars and metabolism. Many of us think that skipping breakfast will be helpful for weight loss, but that certainly isn't the case.

One study looked at women with metabolic syndrome and whether eating more calories in the morning or in the evening was more beneficial for health markers like glucose levels, insulin, and lipids over a twelve-week period. They found that those who ate more calories in the mornings versus in the evening showed greater weight loss and waist circumference reduction, lower levels of fasting glucose and insulin, and a reduction in triglyceride levels by 33.6 percent (Jakubowicz et al. 2013).

A sixteen-year study from Harvard found that male health professionals who regularly skipped breakfast had a 27 percent higher risk for heart attacks and coronary heart disease than the breakfast eaters. They also found that those who skipped breakfast were generally hungrier later in the day and ate more food at night (Cahill 2013). Several other studies have confirmed this as well (Takagi et al. 2019).

Of course, that's not saying eating donuts or cereal for breakfast will help reduce your risk for heart disease. Prioritizing a PFF-balanced breakfast is key. Make sure to check the resource section for some balanced, protein-packed breakfast options.

Eating breakfast in the morning has also been shown to help reduce glucose response after lunch and dinner later in the day. A study found that breakfast skippers showed an impaired insulin response and lower levels of GLP-1, the hormone that enhances insulin secretion (Jakubowicz et al. 2015).

Maybe you're thinking, *But what about all the benefits of intermittent fasting?* There is plenty of research showing the benefits of intermittent fasting, so I'm not ignoring that. Unfortunately, up to 70–75 percent of research studies on intermittent fasting focus on men and not on women. As you probably learned in health education in middle school, men and women are designed very differently, which means that the same benefits intermittent fasting can have on men don't always replicate for women. For example, one study found that intermittent fasting impaired blood sugar regulation for women but not for men (Jakubowicz et al. 2013).

The body also has a better glucose tolerance in the morning than in the evening. A national study found lower fasting glucose and estimated insulin resistance with an earlier eating time in the morning. Often times when someone is skipping breakfast, or following an intermittent fasting sched-ule, they eat more calories later in the day. When it comes to blood sugar support, that's not the best thing (Marriam et al. 2023).

I've seen the power of breakfast in the hundreds of clients I've worked with over the years (as well as myself), so when it comes to blood sugar regulation and overall hormone support, it's a big yes from me.

PREP YOUR BREAKFAST AHEAD OF TIME

I get it, the mornings are hectic and you barely have time to blow-dry your hair, let alone eat breakfast. That's why I always recommend taking some time on the weekends to prep your breakfast ahead of time. Things like egg bakes, overnight oats, or yogurt parfaits take thirty minutes to prep on the weekends and will save you so much time and energy during your week. Check out the simple breakfast recipes in the back of the book starting on page 126.

WHAT IF I'M NOT HUNGRY IN THE MORNING?

One of the most common breakfast questions I get is, "*I don't feel hungry in the morning. Should I still eat breakfast?*" I'm all about listening to your hunger cues, and when it comes to breakfast, this is one time that I say to eat something even if you aren't really hungry. That's because not feeling hungry in the morning can be a result of two things: high levels of stress, or eating a lot right before bedtime. These two can also be related. For example, if you're under a lot of stress, you might not consume the majority of your calories until the evening when you finally have some time to relax.

If you don't really feel hungry in the morning, I would start with a small snack within one hour of waking up. This could be a small apple with some natural peanut butter or a hard-boiled egg with berries. This will help get your body adjusted to eating earlier in the day, which can be helpful for lowering stress, reducing snacking later in the day, improving energy, and changing the distribution of your calories during the entire day.

INCORPORATING INTERMITTENT FASTING IN A BETTER WAY

There's no doubt fasting has its benefits. The human body is not designed for eating all day. With our modern society filled with larger portions, more electronics, and less physical activity, it's important to give the body a break from digesting food. That's why I do recommend a fast of twelve hours overnight. For example, if you normally have breakfast at seven a.m., it's best to avoid eating past seven p.m. This is an easier way to get the benefit of fasting while still getting the benefits of breakfast. According to some researchers, if you fast for over ten hours, the body goes to fat stores for energy, and fatty acids called ketones are released in the bloodstream. This can be helpful for weight loss, as well as protecting memory and learning in the brain (Collier 2013).

Overall, you can have your cake and eat it too (relatively speaking). Get the benefits of breakfast along with the benefits of fasting with a twelve-hour overnight fast.

> **Quick tip:** Eat something in the morning within an hour of waking up to fuel your body and support stable blood sugar levels throughout your day.

CHAPTER 10

PRACTICING MINDFUL EATING

"In order for things to change, we must first be willing to let go of our old ways."

—Ken Keyes Jr.

How many times have you had your lunch while working at your computer, or scrolled on your phone while rushing through your breakfast? Maybe you've sat on the couch to eat your dinner and realized everything on your plate was gone, yet you could barely remember even tasting it. All of these examples are what I call "mindless eating" or "distracted eating," which can contribute to overeating, cravings, and weight gain.

Mindful eating is then defined as *"being present in the moment of eating, appreciating your food, and savoring each bite without distractions."*

The act of eating mindfully has been shown to:

- Improve digestion and absorption of food
- Help reduce cravings
- Increase the enjoyment of eating
- Decrease emotional eating or binge eating
- Increase gratitude about food
- Make healthier and more nourishing food choices

Ultimately, it's not only important to consider what you're eating during the day, but also how you're eating and how food makes you feel. Although socializing with family or friends during a meal can improve your eating experience, answering your emails or scrolling through social media can detract from it.

Studies have found mindful eating to be an effective tool for reducing behaviors like emotional or binge eating, which can be supportive for not just blood sugar balance, but can also support weight and overall diet quality (O'Reilly 2014). For example, I had a client who worked a really fast-paced job in healthcare who started her day with coffee and a granola bar in her car for breakfast. By lunchtime, she was swamped at work and would just get a couple bites in between patients. Once she came home, she was absolutely starving and would raid her kitchen cupboard trying to catch up on her lack of eating earlier in the day. She told me she felt ashamed of her late-night constant snacking but didn't feel like she could stop. It wasn't until she focused on eating more earlier in the day and on blood sugar regulation that her late-night snacking stopped.

HOW TO BE MORE MINDFUL DURING MEALTIME

Put away distractions: Electronics are the number-one distraction at mealtime, whether it's a computer, TV, or phone. The problem with all of these distractions is that it doesn't allow us to be present in the moment of eating and creates stress on our digestion. If you have a desk job where you're sitting in front of a computer, avoid eating your lunch and working at the same time. Not only will your digestion be grateful, but your productivity will improve when you take small breaks during your day. Limiting distractions at mealtimes is especially helpful for distilling healthy mealtime behaviors if you have children. So instead of eating in front of a television or having the tablet out, put all electronics away in a designated spot at mealtime.

Slow down: Being a mom to little kids, I get how sometimes you just want to eat your food quickly while it's still hot and before any milk gets spilt all over the floor. I myself have had to become more mindful about the speed of my eating. But being a fast eater can be stressful on the body, making it more difficult to actually digest and absorb your food well. This can lead to not-so-fun bloating or heartburn later on.

Being a fast eater (which I consider eating a meal in less than twenty minutes) can also lead to overeating at your meal. That's because it takes about twenty minutes for your brain to get the signal that it's full. If you eat your meal in less than twenty minutes, you may still feel hungry, yet your brain just hasn't received the "I'm full" signal yet. So how can you switch your fast eating tendencies to more slower, relaxed ones? An easy trick I use with my clients (and myself) is to put your utensil down between each bite. This automatically forces you to slow down. If you're eating something that doesn't require a utensil, then try to set it down on the plate between each meal and chew your food until it's fully broken down—about apple-sauce consistency.

Ditch the "clean plate" club: Growing up you may have had the "clean plate club" at home or school when it's a goal to clean everything off your plate. Research has found this can be one of the worst things for our eating habits (American Academy of Pediatrics 2014). If you don't like to waste food like me, know that you can always put it in the refrigerator for later. I do this all the time if my kids aren't eating all their food or if I find myself full before all my food is gone. Remember, we don't have to eat all the food on the plate simply because it's there. This can also be helpful when going out to eat. Instead of trying to eat everything on your plate (which is often a lot bigger in portion than we may traditionally have), try putting half of your meal away in a to-go container for later. If you're still hungry after your portion, you can always go back for more.

Check in on your hunger: Everyone was born with their own innate hunger cues, and as we get older those natural hunger cues often get muted. We often eat out of emotion or boredom instead of true hunger. Here's the thing—eating is something we have to do to survive, yet there's often so much emotion tied to it. Taking a minute to check in on your hunger to decide if your desire to eat is because of head hunger (emotional) or phys-ical hunger (you actually need to eat) is going to help you become a more mindful eater. One way to help you check in on your hunger cues before, during, and after meals is using a hunger scale.

The Hunger Scale

1	Starving	6	Satisfied & Light
2	Uncomfortably Hungry	7	Full
3	Very Hungry	8	Very Full
4	A Little Hungry	9	Uncomfortably Full
5	Neutral	10	Painfully Full

Ideally before a meal, you want to be around a three, where you feel hungry but not absolutely starving to the point you could eat anything in sight. After a meal, aim for around seven or eight, where you feel satisfied but you aren't absolutely stuffed like you just ate Thanksgiving dinner.

OTHER THINGS TO FOCUS ON BESIDES THE FOOD'S FLAVOR

Pay attention to how the food looks: We often gravitate toward foods that look good, yet we don't really take the time to pay attention to the small details. For example, what colors do you have on your plate? I encourage incorporating at least three different colors on your plate to get a wide variety of nutrients. Looking at the colors and talking about what they do for our bodies can also be a great teaching tool for children. For example, red foods keep our heart strong, orange foods help us to see, and green foods keep our immune system strong.

Pay attention to how it feels: This can be another great mealtime learning tool. Pay attention to how the food actually feels in your mouth and what texture it is. Is it smooth, crunchy, lumpy, soft, or hard?

Focus on the three F's: If you find yourself struggling with cravings or eating mindlessly out of emotion, one thing that can be helpful is thinking of the three F's: feel, feed, and find.

○ **Feel:** If you have a craving for a particular food (like cookies, for example), ask yourself, *What types of feelings are you experiencing at the moment*? Are you bored? Anxious? Sad? Stressed?

- **Feed:** Then ask yourself, *How does that particular food feed that feeling?* For example, will cookies make you feel less stressed?

- **Find:** Instead of using food (like those cookies) for comfort, what non-food-related behavior can you use to feed the same feeling? For example, if you're feeling stressed, instead of grabbing the sweets in the cabinet, try deep breathing, going for a walk, or calling a friend to vent. Sometimes food is used to give our brains a quick dose of dopamine, yet the effects really don't last very long. Using other things for a source of dopamine can be more helpful and healthier long-term. Listening to music, meditating, moving your body by doing some yoga or going on a walk, and getting some sunlight are some examples.

> **Quick tip:** It's not only important to think about WHAT to eat, but also HOW to eat. Become a more mindful eater by putting away distractions at mealtimes, placing the utensil down between each bite to help you slow down, and doing a check-in on your hunger before, during, and after your meals.

CHAPTER 11

ALL ABOUT HYDRATION

"Your biggest commitment must always be to yourself."
—Bridgett Devoue

"I know I need to drink more water." I hear this almost daily from clients. Maybe you feel the same way because you've heard you should drink eight glasses of water a day. Although that's a general recommendation with little evidence to support it, staying hydrated is essential for your health and your blood sugars.

The human body is made of 60–70 percent water, so without enough water, the body can't do what it's supposed to do. You know you need to drink more H_2O when you struggle with low energy, have dark urine, feel hungry often (because sometimes we feel hungry even though we may just need to hydrate more), have a dry mouth, or experience headaches, muscle aches, and constipation (just to name a few).

Staying hydrated is key for blood sugar balance because it helps reduce glucose spikes from your meals throughout the day. Remember how those spikes can contribute to weight gain, sugar cravings, and low energy? Water helps the kidneys remove excess sugar through urine, which is helpful for lowering blood sugar levels. Low water consumption, on the other hand, can increase the risk for hyperglycemia (or elevated blood sugar levels) (Johnson et al. 2017).

Along with supporting your blood sugars, staying hydrated is key for a number of reasons.

IMPORTANCE OF HYDRATION

Boosting energy and brain function: Low hydration status is linked to a decrease in alertness, fatigue, and confusion. That's because water helps your brain cells communicate with one another and also helps clear out toxins and waste that can impair brain function and energy (Liska et al. 2019).

Supporting your metabolism: Staying hydrated can help you stay full longer and support your metabolism. One specific study looked at the role of drinking excess water and how it impacts weight and body fat reduction for eight weeks. Participants drank about two extra cups of water before each meal (six cups total) above their normal daily water intake. Results found a significant reduction in body weight and body fat compared to pre-study measurements (Vij and Joshi 2013). Overall, drinking water before a meal can be helpful for increasing satiety and reducing overall caloric intake at meals, particularly for adults (Walleghen et al. 2012).

Detoxing the body: Water helps your body excrete waste through sweat, urine, and bowel movements. It also helps the kidneys remove waste from the blood and keep the blood vessels that run to your kidneys clear.

Improving digestion: Water is essential for digestion and absorption of nutrients. About 16 percent of adults, and 33 percent of adults over the age of sixty, struggle with constipation, defined as fewer than three bowel movements a week. Ideally we have a bowel movement daily, and increasing your water intake can be one way to help promote regular daily bowel movements.

Regulating temperature: Water helps regulate the temperature in your body by distributing heat and cooling the body through sweat.

Supporting heart health: Water makes up a large part of the blood, and without enough hydration, your blood can become more concentrated and lead to an imbalance in electrolytes (like sodium and potassium). Electrolytes play a key role in heart health and muscle function. Another bonus—a 2023 study found that optimal water intake can actually help slow the aging process, partly due to the cardiovascular benefits it provides (Dmitrieva et al. 2023).

Improving exercise performance: Low water intake can impact your exercise performance, especially when it comes to high-intensity workouts or exercise in high heat with a lot of sweating. Symptoms like low energy and impaired performance can happen even by losing just 1–2 percent of your body's total water content (Riebel and Davy 2023).

Supporting skin health: The skin is the largest organ, so no wonder water can make a significant difference in how our skin appears. You may notice darker under-eye circles, itchiness, dullness, or more noticeable fine lines when you aren't hydrating enough.

So now that you know the benefits of this inexpensive beverage, let's talk about how to find the right amount for you and how to get more of it.

HOW MUCH WATER SHOULD I DRINK?

As I said earlier, the whole "eight glasses of water a day" is not a supported claim, and that's because everyone's needs are different. Just like everyone needs different amounts of calories, we also need different hydration goals.

A simple way to find how much water you should drink in a day is to take your body weight in pounds and divide it by two. For example, a person who weighs 180 pounds should aim to drink 90 ounces of water each day. Now if you're calculating your number and think that's way more than you drink now, don't worry. As with any change, start out slowly. Maybe right now you have no clue how much water you're drinking, so let's first start tracking to find your starting point. Once you find your starting point, let's see how you can bump it up a bit. For example, if your starting point is forty ounces of water, and your goal is to get to ninety ounces, aim for bumping up your hydration to fifty ounces, then sixty ounces, and so on until you get to your designated goal. Remember, breaking down goals into smaller, more doable steps will make it a lot easier to actually reach your goal.

One of my clients who struggled to drink more water made a simple goal to have a glass of water before each meal. This simple switch helped her bump up her intake by over twenty ounces without even really having to think about it.

Here are other ideas to help you bump up your hydration:

- Pour water into your coffee mug in the morning to help you hydrate before you caffeinate.
- Carry a water bottle with you while running errands, or keep one at your desk at work.
- Set a reminder in your calendar or on your phone to hydrate every hour.
- Fill up water bottles in the morning that equate to the amount of water you need for your day.
- Use reusable straws for your water (sometimes hydrating is just way more fun with a cool straw).
- Enjoy some herbal tea before bed.
- Replace sugary beverages like juice or energy drinks with sparkling water.
- Infuse water with vegetables and fruit like cucumbers, lemon, lime, or frozen berries.
- Try some mineral mocktails made with coconut water (see the recipes in the back of the book).
- Eat foods high in water. Some examples include cucumbers, strawberries, cantaloupe, celery, and zucchini.

IMPORTANCE OF ELECTROLYTES IN WATER

Here's the thing—there's no doubt that increasing your water intake is important. But what often happens when you start drinking more water throughout the day? You'll probably be hanging out more in the bathroom to pee it out. That's why it's important to help your body use the water more effectively through electrolytes.

Electrolytes are minerals like sodium, magnesium, and potassium and are key for helping your body actually absorb all the water you're drinking. This can be as simple as adding a pinch of sea salt to your morning water, putting mineral drops into your water bottle, having unsweetened coconut water (which is a source of potassium), adding electrolyte packets to water, or making mineral mocktails (again, see the recipes in the back of the book). I would try to add some type of electrolyte to your water at least one to two times per day.

WHAT COUNTS AS MY TOTAL WATER INTAKE?

If you're a coffee lover like I am, maybe you're wondering, "*Does coffee count toward my total water intake since it's made with water?*" Unfortunately, no. I suggest only counting non-caffeinated beverages as part of your water intake since caffeinated beverages can act as a diuretic. Non-caffeinated beverages could include herbal teas, sparkling waters, infused water, or electrolyte mixtures.

> **Quick tip:** Drinking half your body weight in ounces of water throughout the day will help you stay hydrated and support blood sugars. Include some electrolytes to help your body use the water more effectively.

CHAPTER 12

NAVIGATING NUTRITION LABELS AND GROCERY SHOPPING

"What you do every day matters more than what you do once in a while."

—Gretchen Rubin

Have you ever gone down an aisle at the grocery store, looked at all the options available, felt instant overwhelm, and had no clue what to even look for on the food products? If so, this chapter is for you.

Grocery stores are laid out in a very strategic way to help increase buying behavior. For example, produce is often displayed in the front to represent a "fresh" environment, whereas staples like milk and eggs are displayed in the back to force you to walk past several other products. Along with the layout of a typical grocery store, products are also placed in strategic ways. For example, the more expensive products are at eye-level versus the generic versions at the bottom.

Food companies also use certain language to help entice you to buy their product. Terms like "fat-free," "heart healthy," or "low cholesterol" can often be found on the front of a food product. As discussed in Chapter 5, simply trusting what the front of a food product says doesn't give you the whole picture. It's important to turn the food product over and become your own investigator to see what ingredients are actually in the product.

I showed you a nutrition facts label in Chapter 8 when we talked about sugar, and along with looking at the "added sugar" in a product, let's walk through some other parts of the label to keep your eye on.

Calories: Simply looking at the calorie count doesn't give you the whole picture, but it is helpful to pay attention to calories per serving size. For example, a single serving size (twelve chips) of Doritos has about 150 calories, but there are fifteen servings in one bag. Just say you have three servings (or thirty-six chips) because you're munching on them while watching your favorite movie; the calories consumed go up to 450 calories. Calories can add up quickly if we're mindlessly eating and not paying attention to servings.

Fat: I've mentioned before that we don't need to fear all fat because it really depends on the *quality* of the fat. One area when it comes to the fat section is to pay attention to "trans fats" because these are the most harmful type of fat and should be avoided completely. Remember to pay attention to words like "*partially hydrogenated*" or "*hydrogenated oils*" under the ingredient list because those are other names for trans fats.

Sodium: This mineral often gets a bad reputation, but just like fats, it depends on the quality. Sodium is an essential electrolyte; we could literally die without it. I'm all about adding some sea salt to my cooking to help enhance flavor. Sodium becomes a problem, though, when the foods you're consuming are mainly processed foods with a lot of added sodium in them to help extend their shelf-life. If a product contains a high level of sodium (over 20 percent), it's best to put it back on the shelf.

Carbohydrates: You're now an expert at knowing carbohydrates can raise your blood sugar, and when it comes to this section, it's important to pay attention to the fiber (which will help lower your blood sugar) and added sugar (which will raise your blood sugar). Generally, I recommend aiming for at least five grams of fiber per serving and under ten grams of added sugar per serving.

Protein: if you're using something like Greek yogurt or a protein powder, be sure to check the protein. I generally recommend aiming for at least twenty grams of protein at meals and about ten grams at snacks.

Micronutrients: You'll see on the bottom of the nutrition facts label that certain micronutrients, like vitamin D and iron, are highlighted. Although there are no specific guidelines for how much to get in each product, I always look at whether a particular food item is a good source of any of those. Vitamin D, calcium, and potassium in particular are key players in supporting optimal blood sugars.

Ingredients: Last but not least, I encourage you to be your own investigator and look at the ingredients. Simply just relying on what the front of the label says does not give us the whole picture. Look at the top five ingredients in the product to see what it contains the most of. When in doubt, if it sounds like it contains ingredients that would be used in a science experiment, I'd put it back on the shelf.

Some common ingredients to avoid in products:

- Partially hydrogenated or hydrogenated oils (aka trans fats)
- High fructose corn syrup
- Refined oils like vegetable, canola, or soybean
- Sodium nitrates
- Artificial sweeteners like aspartame or sucralose
- Monosodium glutamate
- Artificial flavors and colors like blue #1, red #3, or yellow #6

TRICKS TO USE WHEN READING A NUTRITION LABEL

Here are two tricks I use when reviewing nutrition facts labels to quickly make more informed decisions on products.

FIVE-TO-ONE RATIO FOR CARBS AND FIBER

Fiber is your friend for balancing your blood sugar, and oftentimes products are low in fiber but high in carbohydrates overall. So aiming for a five-to-one ratio for carbs and fiber is helpful for bumping up your fiber intake.

How to do it: Divide the amount of carbs by fiber and aim for that number to be less than five. For example, if a product has 14 grams of carbohydrates and 3 grams of fiber, you would divide 14 by 3, which equates to 4.6. Since 4.6 is less than 5, this product would fit into that ratio.

PROTEIN + FIBER > SUGAR

I've talked about the importance of fiber for blood sugar regulation, but protein is also a huge part of the team as well. With this trick, you simply add up the amount of protein and fiber in a food product and aim for that number to be more than the total sugar amount.

How to do it: For example, let's say a product has 9 grams of protein, 3 grams of fiber, and 15 grams of sugar. The amount of sugar is more than the amount of protein and fiber combined (9 + 3 = 12), so that would not be the best option.

I know going to the grocery store and being bombarded with clever food marketing can feel overwhelming. Get a free printable grocery shopping list and pantry essentials list at https://autumnenloe.com/bloodsugarbook.

"BUT HEALTHY FOOD IS EXPENSIVE."

If you're like most people, you've probably felt this way before. Sure, you can go through the fast food drive-thru and order off the dollar menu, but is that type of food going to fuel your health long-term? I like to give the analogy of our health as a bank. We are either depositing nourishing food into the bank or withdrawing from our bank with poor, processed, low-nutrient-dense foods. We are either paying for our health now by eating good-quality, nutrient-dense foods or paying for our health later with complications. Poor nutrition is the number-one cause of death and disease. I personally would rather put more of an investment into good nutrition now versus paying for medical bills later. And that's not even taking into account how the quality of your life can change by prioritizing high-quality foods. Energy, digestion, cravings, mental health, and overall confidence are directly tied to the quality of foods you eat each day.

Plus, cooking real, wholesome food at home can actually be cheaper in the long run. The average cost of a restaurant meal is thirteen dollars. The average cost of a home-cooked meal? Just four dollars. When you focus more on cooking at home, and less on take-out, you can actually save money over time.

Let's dive into how to save money on food by cooking more at home in the next chapter.

CHAPTER 13

· · · · · · · · · ·

MASTERING MEAL PREP

"It's no coincidence that four of the six letters in health are heal."

—Ed Northstrum

Meal prepping is often thought of as spending hours in the kitchen on a Sunday prepping meals for your busy week ahead. Although that may be how some people do it, I have some strategies to help you simplify meal prep without spending hours in the kitchen (or losing your sanity).

Why are we talking about meal prepping in the first place? To start, having a plan for your meals can be a game-changer for your health. How often have you gone through the drive-thru or ordered take-out after a long day of work, because you had no idea what to make for dinner? Taking some time on the weekends to plan your meals for the upcoming week helps you start your week on a healthy note, saves you time later on, and is also better for your bank account. Yes, it takes some time initially, especially as you're getting into a groove. After some practice though, I know you'll become a meal-prepping pro.

THE 1-2-3 METHOD FOR MEAL PREPPING

A simple method I teach my clients to help them simplify meal prepping is called the "1-2-3 method" for meal prepping. This simple method helps you plan your meals for your upcoming week and prevents food waste (while also saving you money!). You can also switch it up as you'd like, depending on your family size and meal preference.

The 1-2-3 method for meal prepping includes:

○ **1—one main breakfast meal that you can switch up throughout the week.** For example, if you make an egg bake, you can switch up the types of sides you have with it. Or if you're making yogurt parfaits, you can switch up the toppings.

○ **2—two lunches that you alternate.** For example, you can alternate between salad or soups, or make turkey wraps for part of the week and tuna salad for the remaining days.

○ **3—three main dinners for your week (includes leftovers).** This involves alternating between three main dinners and their leftovers. This may involve doubling recipes as needed. Depending on your family size, this may look more like having four main meals. As with the others, you can switch it up to prevent boredom. For example, if you made tacos one night, you could do a quesadilla night with the leftovers.

When you base your meals using the 1-2-3 method, it becomes a lot easier to plan your meals for the week. I typically use the 1-2-3 method for the weekdays since the weekends provide more time to cook different foods.

EXAMPLE OF MEALS USING THE 1-2-3 METHOD FOR THE WEEKDAYS

	Breakfast	Lunch	Dinner
Day 1	Egg bake with an orange and almonds on the side	White chicken chili with veggies and dip	Taco night
Day 2	Egg bake with avocado slices and an apple	White chicken chili with veggies and dip	Taco night
Day 3	Egg bake with an orange and almonds on the side	White chicken chili with veggies and dip	Egg roll bowl

EXAMPLE OF MEALS USING THE 1-2-3 METHOD FOR THE WEEKDAYS

	Breakfast	Lunch	Dinner
Day 4	Egg bake with avocado slices and an apple	Turkey wraps with a Caesar salad	Egg roll bowl
Day 5	Egg bake with an orange and almonds on the side	Turkey wraps with a Caesar salad	Sheet-pan chicken and veggies

You can switch up the 1-2-3 method to fit your family size and needs. For example, maybe you do a 2-2-4 method, or a 1-3-5 method. Find what works for you and your family.

WHAT TO PRIORITIZE FOR MEAL PREPPING

Before I plan out any meals for the week, I first take inventory of the foods I already have on hand. Have some extra eggs? Make an egg bake. Have some tuna in the cupboard you want to use up? Make a tuna salad for lunch. After that, I write down the food items I still need to get and make a shopping list from there.

Although you can certainly cook all the foods ahead of time, there's definitely no need to do that. There are a couple things I would prep ahead of time though, and that includes your breakfast and lunches if you work outside the home or don't have a lot of time to prep lunches. Having a breakfast option prepped ahead of time can make the hectic mornings go so much more smoothly. How many times have you grabbed something quick, like a granola bar or just nothing at all because you ran out of time to have breakfast in the morning? Things like egg bakes, yogurt parfaits, oatmeal bakes, bags for your smoothie ingredients, or a batch of hard-boiled eggs can take less than an hour to prep and saves so much time and energy during the week.

BUILDING BALANCED MEALS

We talked a lot about building PFF-balanced meals in Chapter 5, so how can you create these balanced meals while meal prepping?

Here's a simple strategy:

○ **Start with your protein:** such as eggs, cottage cheese, Greek yogurt, beef, rotisserie chicken, or fish

○ **Add some fibrous veggies and/or fruit:** such as sliced bell peppers, carrots, cucumbers, broccoli, salad greens, berries, or sliced apples

○ **Add some nourishing fat:** including nuts, avocado slices, olives, nut butter, or cooking oils like avocado or coconut oil

After that, fill in the rest, whether you want to add noodles, rice, or sourdough bread. Prioritizing PFF first will help ensure a balanced and nourishing meal every time. And remember, eating your protein first at your meal before starchier carbohydrates like bread or pasta will help improve blood sugar levels.

BATCH COOKING

Another thing that can make the world of meal prepping a lot easier is batch cooking. This is essentially making large batches of food to use in different meals throughout the week. For example, you could make a bunch of chicken breasts to use in various ways—as a protein on top of a salad or for chicken tortilla soup at dinner. Another example would be dicing up several zucchinis to use for a stir fry at dinner, in smoothies at breakfast, and as a dipper for tuna salad at lunch. Making a large batch of certain food items and incorporating them in several different ways can save a lot of time, energy, and money, let alone help keep food from getting moldy in the fridge.

HACKS TO KEEP PRODUCE LASTING LONGER

Speaking of moldy food, let's talk about ways to help keep fresh produce lasting longer *(because how proud do you feel when you actually finish the whole box of spinach before it gets all slimy?)*. If you're investing the time and money into buying real, nutrient-dense foods, I'm sure you don't want to just end up throwing them in the garbage, or having them get smelly in the back of your fridge.

Here are some "hacks" that I like to use to help food last longer:

○ Soak wilted veggies in water to crisp them up (this is great for celery).

○ Keep mushrooms in a paper bag to help prevent them from getting slimy.

○ Keep avocados in the fridge to help prevent them ripening quickly.

○ Add cucumbers that are about to go bad to water to flavor it.

○ Store berries in a mason jar with a lid to keep them fresh longer.

○ Blend spinach that's about to go bad with water, and pour it into ice cube trays. Simply remove the ice cubes and add them to sauces or smoothies.

○ Store potatoes in a cool, dry place away from other produce.

○ Wash banana stems to prevent fruit flies, and store overripe bananas in the freezer to use later.

> **Quick tip:** Getting into a rhythm with meal prepping can take some time to make it a habit. Start out by setting twenty minutes on the weekends to plan out your meals for your upcoming week, and go from there. It's worth it. I promise!

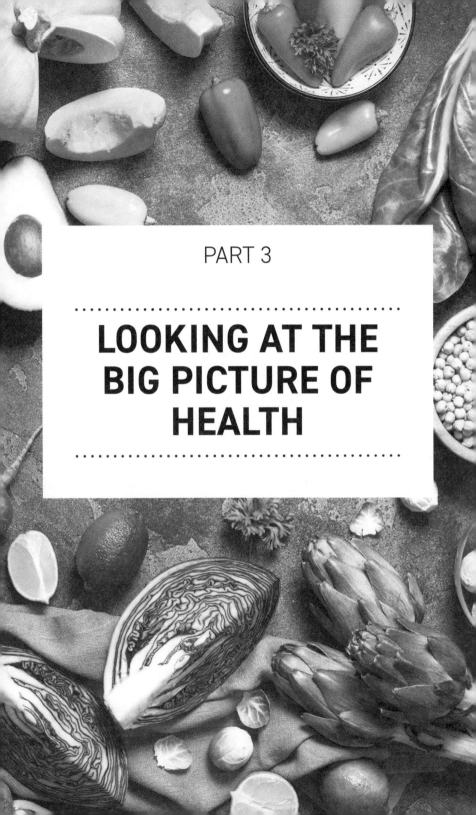

PART 3

LOOKING AT THE BIG PICTURE OF HEALTH

CHAPTER 14

THE LINK BETWEEN CORTISOL AND BLOOD SUGAR

"The power for creating a better future is contained in the present moment: You create a good future by creating a good present."

—Eckhart Tolle

"I've gained forty pounds since starting this job." My client Lucy was explaining the reason she was seeking help with her nutrition. She was working really long hours, and would come home after her exhausting day and automatically go to food to help her cope with all the stress.

Unfortunately, this case is not uncommon. If I were to ask you if you had some type of stress in your life, I'm guessing the answer would be, *"Of course!"* We all experience some form of stress, whether it's from a stressful job, relationships, illness, or just figuring out what to make for dinner; all of these are forms of stress—whether big or small, and they all add up.

Stress can also occur from:

- Not eating enough or eating too much during the day
- Blood sugar dysregulation
- A lack of breaks
- Too much exposure to electronics
- A lack of sleep/not getting high-quality sleep
- Overexercising
- Lack of exercise
- Clutter
- Endocrine disruptors from body, skincare, and cleaning products

I get that stress isn't the most interesting topic to talk about, but stress is the culprit of all our health struggles in some shape or form. Like my client Lucy, I find many people don't prioritize stress management until they've reached burnout, can't sleep at night, or discover their clothes are starting to feel too tight. We can't just wait until we're overwhelmed and burnt out to lower stress in the body; it needs to be a daily practice.

Data from the American Psychological Association shows that stress levels (especially since the COVID-19 pandemic) have increased in adults, with almost 60 percent claiming to feel more stressed out. Work stress can be a huge culprit of this, with 83 percent of workers in the United States reporting work-related stress, and 54 percent claiming that work stress affects their home life (US Department of Labor n.d.). How many times have you gone home from a stressful day at work and felt more short-tempered with your family or stress-ate through your kitchen cupboard?

Although some stress is actually good for us and can help us perform daily activities, the problem is when it becomes chronic and unmanaged. Maybe you're the way I used to be and only really think of stress management when getting a massage or taking a bubble bath once in a while. It was always on the back burner. As a former perfectionist with a type A personality, I used to gravitate toward stress without realizing it. The more busy I was, the more accomplished I felt. And this is common in our modern-day culture. What's the most popular response we hear when we ask someone how they are? Typically it's "*busy!*" Of course being busy can be a good thing in some capacity, but our schedules are continuously filled up, and feeling stressed out and overwhelmed is the norm. From my personal experience, all that "wearing busy as a badge of honor" took a toll on my health, and I started taking stress management way more seriously.

Although I'm all about massages and bubble baths to help feel calm and relaxed, there are things we can do on a daily basis with very limited effort that can have a huge impact on our overall stress levels.

But first, let's dive into a powerful hormone: cortisol.

CORTISOL 101

When we experience stress, the adrenal glands produce both cortisol and adrenaline. Together, these two hormones work together in what we call the "fight-or-flight" response—a reaction to a stressful or dangerous situation. For thousands of years, these two hormones helped protect our ancestors from predators. Nowadays though, many of us are living in "fight-or-flight" mode, and it's leading to an increase in blood pressure and belly fat, negatively impacting immunity, damaging the brain's memory center, and contributing to poor blood sugar regulation. Yes, you're going to have to deal with stress on a regular basis; the problem arises when it's left there untreated.

For example, you have to deal with a stressful mishap at work. Just because you dealt with that particular stressful event at the moment *doesn't mean you actually dealt with the stress you felt from it*. Oftentimes, the stressors we endure all day long get piled up like a huge pile of laundry waiting to get folded.

Cortisol is a steroid hormone and is synthesized by cholesterol. It affects nearly every organ system in the body, from the nervous system, to the cardiovascular, to the reproductive, to the immune system.

Cortisol plays a variety of functions in the body, including

- Helping the body respond to stress or danger (for example, giving you a burst of energy if you had to run away from danger).
- Helping regulate the circadian rhythm. Cortisol is highest in the morning to give your body energy and wake you up, and then it gradually reduces throughout the day. It's lowest in the evening before bed to help your body wind down and go to sleep.
- In a healthy state, adjusting your metabolism and supporting your immunity.

One of cortisol's superpowers is to help the body have enough energy to get through a stressful situation. It will rise to help prompt the liver to release a stored form of glucose called glycogen into the bloodstream for energy. Simply put, it helps increase blood glucose levels so you have energy to respond to a stressor. For example, if you skip a meal, cortisol can raise blood glucose levels. When this happens, your pancreas also produces more insulin (the fat-storage hormone) to get your rising blood glucose levels back to normal. Although this is a great example of how the human body is there to work for you and support you, it's obviously not ideal to rely on cortisol to balance glucose levels. If your body is constantly having to pump out cortisol to balance your blood glucose levels, and insulin is also getting pumped out all the time, this can lead to a host of health problems, including increasing your risk for insulin resistance and diabetes.

So although cortisol has some benefits, we want to avoid too high or too low levels of cortisol.

Signs of elevated cortisol:
- Weight gain, especially around the midsection
- High blood pressure
- Trouble falling asleep
- Anxiety or depression
- Digestive issues like constipation or diarrhea
- Irritability
- Difficulty concentrating
- Cravings
- Headaches

Opposite of that, we can also experience low cortisol. This can happen if levels of cortisol are continuously elevated, leaving the body the inability to produce cortisol at a level it should be.

Signs of low cortisol:
- Weight loss
- Low blood pressure
- Morning sluggishness
- Weakened immunity
- Anxiety or depression
- Cravings
- Loss of resilience during stress

STRATEGIES TO REDUCE STRESS

We all experience stress, and whether you have just a couple of the symptoms listed above or a lot of them, it's important to prioritize some type of stress reduction every single day. Your health and blood sugars literally depend on it. Here are some ideas.

Identifying your stressors: In general, there are two types of stress: physical and mental. Physical stress can be a result of our diet, exercise, or sleep habits. Mental stressors can happen from things like work, relationships, or home life. Although there's some stress we can't eliminate entirely, it can be helpful to make a list of all your physical and mental stressors. Take that list and look at ones that can be reduced or eliminated. Maybe that means doing grocery delivery to help save time or getting up ten minutes earlier in the morning so you don't feel so rushed out the door.

Prioritizing real, wholesome foods: Your eating habits can have a huge impact on how your body deals with stress. Food is the body's fuel, and when we're not fueling the body enough, or fueling it with refined, low-nutrient foods, it's going to cause more stress on the body. Instead, prioritize real foods that come from animals or plants instead of man-made ingredients. Think of eggs for breakfast instead of cereal, or snacking on carrots with nuts instead of chips. The body isn't designed to digest preservatives and other artificial ingredients. We truly are what we eat, and when you focus on foods in their most natural state, they're a lot more usable in the body and will help lower stress versus raising it.

Short on time to prepare meals? Keep it simple with the 1-2-3 method described in the previous chapter.

Practicing meditation: Although meditation has been around for thousands of years, it's become more popular in the present years as a way to cope with stress. That's because meditation activates the body's relaxation response, which lowers the production of cortisol. It can also help reduce the release of inflammation in the body. For example, one study looking at the benefits of an eight-week mindfulness-based stress reduction practice found a reduction in the inflammatory chemicals called cytokines in study participants (which are released with an increase in cortisol) (Rosenkranz 2013). Meditation doesn't need to take a lot of time; even a couple minutes of becoming mindful of your breath can be helpful. For example, inhale for the count of four, hold for the count of five, and exhale for the count of six. This can easily be done in the car or shower.

Moving your body: When you think of exercise, what first comes to mind? For some people, they dread exercise or simply feel they don't have time for it (especially when you're so busy feeling stressed!). As someone who used to do a lot of cardio despite absolutely dreading it, I'm here to tell you, exercise does not have to mean spending an hour at the gym or doing burpees in your basement. In fact, when you're under a lot of stress, doing a lot of cardio can actually wreak havoc on your hormones versus help them. The goal with movement is to get the hormone and blood sugar benefits without causing more stress on the body. Focus on incorporating some type of movement that you enjoy for at least thirty minutes a day (this can also be broken down into smaller segments if that works better for you). I'll be diving more into this in Chapter 16.

Supporting your gut: Stress can impact the health of your gut by decreasing gastric secretion, motility, and its barrier function, thus making you experience digestive issues and a suppressed immune system. If you've ever found differences in your bowel movements under stress, whether it's constipation or the urge to go more often, this is why. Stress can also decrease your feel-good neurotransmitters (like serotonin) which help calm your body during times of stress. We'll dive more into supporting your gut in the next chapter.

Prioritizing sleep: According to the American Psychological Association, adults who get fewer than eight hours of sleep a night are more likely to report feeling more stressed. Sleep is the time for your body to recharge, and when we don't get enough of it, it can lead to damage later on (American Psychological Association 2024). If stress is causing you to not sleep well at night, Chapter 17 is for you.

Giving thanks: Practicing gratitude may be the last thing you want to do when you're feeling stressed, and at the same time, it can be a powerful tool to alleviate stress. That's because practicing gratitude releases two crucial neurotransmitters from the brain called dopamine and serotonin, which are responsible for emotions and making you feel good. I like to think of five things I'm grateful for every morning while I'm getting ready for the day. Whether you're practicing gratitude for something big, like your home, or something small, like a really good cup of tea, focusing on the good will help you notice more of the good during your day. If you struggle with thinking of things to be grateful for in the present moment, you could think of someone in your life you're grateful for instead. Another trick to try is to change the words "I have to" to "I get to." For example, "I get to make dinner" versus "I have to make dinner." Although things like dishes and laundry are definitely not on my favorites list, changing how I talk about them makes doing them a little easier.

Regulating the nervous system: Your nervous system is your body's command center, and incorporating certain techniques to help regulate it can help your body get out of the "fight-or-flight" response during stress. Some examples to help regulate your nervous system at home include: spending time in nature, incorporating grounding exercises (like walking barefoot on the grass), dancing, deep breathing, going on a walk, singing and humming, lying down with your legs up the wall, or using weighted blankets.

Watching your sugar intake: We dove deep into sugar in Chapter 8, and although it's easy to grab a Snickers bar in times of stress, too much sugar intake can impair the body's ability to cope with stress, let alone the blood sugar spikes that it can create, which, as you know, causes even *more* stress on the body. Take a breath when you have an urge to grab sugary foods when you're feeling stressed, and remember, blood sugar regulation is essential during times of stress.

Auditing your caffeine consumption: Caffeine is a stimulant, which means it can trigger the "fight-or-flight" response in the body and increase cortisol levels in the body. Although I'm all about a good cup of coffee in the morning, it's important to be mindful about how much you're having throughout the day. Limit caffeine intake to no more than 200 milligrams (or two cups of coffee) per day. Keep in mind, two cups of coffee doesn't mean two cups in a huge fifteen-ounce coffee mug from Target; it means a true coffee cup size, which is about eight to ten ounces. Also, when it comes to your morning cup of coffee, aim to fuel your body first before you caffeinate (hydrate and fuel before you caffeinate), and limit caffeine after noon so it doesn't impact your sleep.

USING FOOD TO LOWER STRESS IN THE BODY

Certain foods can be a helpful tool to lower stress in the body. Some of those include:

Antioxidants: These protect your cells against free radicals, which are molecules produced when your body is under stress. Certain foods are particularly high in antioxidants, including berries (of any kind), kale, extra-virgin olive oil, cherries, salmon, chia seeds, and mushrooms.

Vitamin C: Commonly known for its immunity benefits, it also has been shown to support the body with stress. In fact, the adrenal glands use up vitamin C at a more rapid rate during times of stress (National Institutes of Health 2021). Sources of vitamin C include oranges, grapefruit, kiwi, strawberries, bell peppers, broccoli, and brussels sprouts.

Protein: This macronutrient is one that your body needs even more during times of stress. That's because amino acids from proteins make up the hormones and neurotransmitters that create your body's stress response. Protein is also great for keeping you feeling full, balancing blood sugars, and reducing sugar cravings, which can increase during times of stress. Prioritize a source of protein at every meal and snack.

Omega-3s: These are a group of three important fats: ALA, DHA, and EPA, which have been shown to reduce stress and inflammation in the body. Along with that, they can help reduce early aging and mortality, reduce hyperlipidemia and hypertension, and slow the buildup of plaque, which can block arteries (Madison et al. 2021). Sources of Omega-3s include salmon, sardines, flaxseeds, chia seeds, and walnuts.

Probiotics: These are live microorganisms that help to fuel the good bacteria in the gut, which can become imbalanced during times of stress. Sources of natural probiotics include Greek yogurt, kefir, kimchi, miso, raw sauerkraut, fermented vegetables, and kombucha.

SUPPLEMENTS TO HELP SUPPORT STRESS

Along with food, there are certain supplements that can be supportive during stressful times. Some of those include:

Prebiotics & probiotics: Along with getting prebiotics and probiotics from food (discussed in the next chapter), adding a daily probiotic supplement containing the two during times of stress can be helpful to support your gut health. Probiotics are live microorganisms that support the beneficial bacteria in the gut, and prebiotics are the food for the probiotics. Look for a supplement with several strains, such as *Lactobacillus* and *Bifidobacterium*, and one that contains a minimum of five billion CFU (colony-forming units).

L-theanine: This is an amino acid that can help you feel more calm and relaxed. The calming effects of L-theanine usually kick in within about thirty to sixty minutes after taking it, and it is best absorbed with caffeine. General dosage: 100–400 milligrams/day. Along with supplement form, it can also be found in green tea and matcha tea. (Check out the iced coconut matcha latte recipe in the back of the book.)

Adaptogens: These are made of herbs or other plant substances (like mushrooms) that can help the body manage and lower stress in the body. You can find adaptogens in several different forms, including ashwagandha, ginseng, reishi, rhodiola, and holy basil.

Magnesium: As discussed in Chapter 7, this is one of my favorite minerals (and supplements) of all. The body needs more magnesium during times of stress, and since many people are lacking in this important mineral, it can be a helpful one to add during times of stress. Bonus—it's a muscle relaxant, so it can be helpful for winding down the body before bed and suppressing the release of cortisol. General dosage: 200–400 milligrams.

WHAT TO CONSIDER BEFORE TAKING SUPPLEMENTS

Prioritize food first: Supplements are there to fill in the gaps that diet alone isn't filling, or that your body needs more of during a particular time. Supplements should never be used to replace food though. Simply said, supplements are most effective in conjunction with healthy eating habits.

They can interfere with medications: It's important to know that certain supplements can interfere with some medications. For example, holy basil can lower the effectiveness of thyroid hormone medications. Always check with your healthcare provider before trying a new supplement.

They aren't for everyone: Certain supplements may not be appropriate for certain populations. For example, ashwagandha should be avoided if you have an autoimmune disease or are pregnant.

The supplement industry is poorly regulated: Supplements are not regulated in the same way medications are. You can go to most retail stores and find supplements on the shelves. Since it is a poorly regulated industry, I recommend always making sure the supplements you take are tested by a third party. This means an outside party is testing the supplement for quality, potency, and purity. This not only helps improve the safety of the supplement, it will also improve the effectiveness and save you from wasting money on supplements that are of poor quality.

More isn't always better: I've had clients tell me they're taking twenty different supplements without really knowing the purpose of each one. Know that more isn't always better, and it's important to know why you're taking the supplements in the first place.

Get my free supplement guide for stress with brand links at https://autumnenloe.com/bloodsugarbook.

> **Quick tip:** It's important to note that you don't want to stress yourself out by trying to reduce stress. Pick one to two things you can realistically do daily to support your body with stress.

CHAPTER 15

• • • • • • • • • • • •

WHAT'S YOUR GUT HAVE TO DO WITH IT?

"The gut is a garden, requiring care and nourishment to thrive."

—Giulia Enders

I've been talking about gut health throughout this book so far, and although it's a topic that's becoming more popular, it's still an area that is often overlooked in our modern healthcare system. It's an essential part of your health and when it comes to blood sugars, your gut has a lot to do with it.

GUT HEALTH 101

Most people think of gut health in terms of just digestion, but it's so much more than that. Your gut is composed of over one hundred trillion bacteria that make up what is called the *gut microbiome.* A healthy gut environment means there's the right balance between the good (helpful) and bad (potentially harmful) bacteria. Within the first few days of life, the gut environment is colonized with bacteria and continues to change and adapt throughout your life. The foods you eat, stress levels, and sleep are some of the many contributors to the health of your gut. Conditions like constipation, allergies, autoimmunity, inflammatory bowel disease, obesity, diabetes, and poor immunity can all be tied back to gut health, and it's estimated that sixty to seventy million people are affected by some type of digestive disorder (National Institute of Diabetes and Digestive and Kidney Diseases 2014).

There are a lot of factors that go into the health of your gut, including your age, nutrition, medication use (especially the use of antibiotics), genetics, exercise, toxin exposure, and hygiene. (Did you know it's actually possible to be too clean?)

Not only are there different types of bacteria in the gut, there's also an intestinal barrier to help protect it. It's like a security guard to prevent pathogens and bacteria from entering the party. This intestinal barrier is made of a single layer of epithelial cells (just one!). That means when the intestinal barrier becomes deteriorated (from things like stress, poor sleep, or low-nutrient-dense foods), it increases the risk for a condition called "leaky gut" that's associated with disorders like inflammatory bowel disease, nonalcoholic fatty liver disease, obesity, fibromyalgia, allergies, and diabetes (Aleman et al. 2023).

THE GUT PLAYS A VITAL ROLE IN YOUR HEALTH

Not only does a healthy gut environment help improve your digestion, it's also the site where 90 percent of serotonin is produced (which helps us to stress less and feel more relaxed and calm), it contains 70–80 percent of the immune system, it's the place where vitamins like B vitamins, vitamin K, and amino acids are produced, it regulates the metabolism, and it's the site where absorption of food takes place.

There's also a constant connection between your gut and brain. In fact, the gut is considered the second brain. That's why improving the health of your gut can also positively impact moods and motivation.

Without a healthy gut environment, several areas of your health can be negatively impacted, such as:

- Your mental health
- Thyroid health
- Immunity
- Metabolism and energy levels
- Skin health
- Hormone health
- Absorption of nutrients

And when it comes to your blood sugars, the health of your gut is also tied to that too.

YOUR GUT AND BLOOD SUGARS

When blood glucose levels are imbalanced, it can impact the type of bacteria present in the gut. With hyperglycemia, for example, the intestinal barrier becomes disrupted and alters the type of gut bacteria present. When this happens (also known as dysbiosis), it increases the risk for inflammation, obesity, metabolic syndrome, and type 2 diabetes (Aishwarya Sadagopan et al. 2023, Oana Iatcu et al. 2022).

Artificial sweeteners can also alter the gut bacteria. A study in 2022 found that participants who consumed artificial sweeteners for two weeks had an altered gut microbiome and elevated blood glucose levels (Scientific American 2022). *See why artificial sweeteners aren't so sweet after all?*

Elevated glucose levels can also increase the risk for infection. This is because bacteria thrive on excess sugar in the bloodstream and keep immune cells from doing what they need to do to prevent infection (Berbudi et al. 2020).

Supporting your gut isn't something to just focus on if you have to take an antibiotic or you're feeling constipated. It's an area that should be part of your day-to-day life since it has such a powerful influence on overall health.

Signs your gut needs some extra support:

- Digestive issues like gas, constipation, diarrhea, heartburn or bloating
- Sugar cravings
- Unintentional weight changes
- Sleep disturbances or fatigue
- Food intolerances
- High frequency of sickness (like getting a cold)
- Low moods or anxiety
- Skin issues like acne or eczema
- Autoimmunity
- Imbalanced blood sugars
- Headaches/migraines
- Obesity
- Reflux

WAYS TO SUPPORT YOUR GUT HEALTH

Now that you know why the gut is such a big deal, let's talk about ways to support it through your food and lifestyle habits.

START WITH FOOD

Add in probiotic-rich foods and beverages: These help to fuel the good bacteria in the gut.
Sources include: plain Greek yogurt, raw sauerkraut, apple cider vinegar, miso, kimchi, kombucha, and kefir.

Incorporate prebiotic-rich foods: These are food for probiotics.
Sources include: bananas, apples, avocados, onions, garlic leeks, artichokes, jicama, asparagus, oats, and flaxseed.

Make sure you're eating enough fiber: Along with probiotics, fiber also helps provide nourishment to the good bacteria. Aim for at least twenty-five to thirty grams of fiber each day.
Sources include: avocados, beans, oats, raspberries, artichokes, lentils, and peas.

Add in bitters: Bitters have been used for thousands of years to support digestion by stimulating the flow of digestive juices.
Sources include: radicchio, cruciferous vegetables, ginger, arugula, artichokes, bitter melon, green tea, coffee, dandelion, grapefruit, cranberries, turmeric, and cocoa.

Incorporate diversity: The diet of most Americans is pretty colorless. This wreaks havoc on the gut because the gut microbiome thrives on having a diversity of foods. An easy way to incorporate more diversity at meals is to aim for at least three different colors on your plate, and try not to eat the same foods all the time. For example, if you love a morning smoothie for breakfast, switch up the types of fruit and vegetables you're putting in it.

Focus on nourishing fats: Research has found a high-fat "Western-style" diet increases the relative abundance of bad bacteria at the expense of good bacteria (Davis 2017). Focus on nourishing fats, including avocados, extra-virgin olive oil, and plain nuts and seeds versus foods made with trans fats, canola, vegetable, or soybean oil.

Limit added sugar consumption: Excess sugar intake can feed the not-so-great bacteria in the gut, along with increasing your glucose levels. Pay attention to added sugar content in your foods by looking at the "added sugar" section on a nutrition label. Chapter 8 talks about this in detail.

ASSESS YOUR DAILY HABITS

Along with food, certain lifestyle habits can also influence the makeup of your gut, including:

Stress: Although we just talked about stress in the previous chapter, it's important to mention it here because it can directly impact gut health as well. For example, when you're under stress you may notice differences in your digestion, hunger, or moods. Find something you can implement daily to help your body manage stress.

Sleep: Not only does a lack of sleep negatively impact your energy levels, it also literally changes the type of bacteria found in your gut. For example, studies have found that sleep deprivation and shift-work changes your gene expression and the makeup of the bacteria in the gut (Yuanyuan et al. 2018). Stay tuned for more about sleep in Chapter 17.

Hydration: Staying well hydrated not only helps prevent issues like constipation, it can also enhance bacterial diversity in the gut. It's also important to consider the source and quality of your water. Drinking-water sources are ranked among the key contributing factors of gut bacteria variation (Vanhaecke et al. 2022).

Exercise: Studies have found that exercise can increase the number of beneficial bacteria, along with enriching the diversity of bacteria. Plus, exercise can help lower blood sugar levels. Aim for thirty minutes of some type of exercise each day.

How fast you're eating: Eating too quickly can impact how well your food is digested and absorbed. Focus on slowing down while you eat by putting your utensil down between each bite and taking three deep breaths before each meal to help relax the body. Remember, it's hard to digest if your body is stressed.

As you can see, your gut does so much more than simply digesting your food. And when it comes to your blood sugars, your gut really does have a lot to do with it.

> **Quick tip:** Nourish your gut every single day by eating foods high in fiber, prebiotics, and probiotics; including diversity in your meals; and taking three deep breaths before each meal to improve digestion.

CHAPTER 16

• • • • • • • • • • • •

MOVEMENT IS MEDICINE

"It's not whether you 'feel' like putting in the work, but whether or not you do it regardless."

—Brianna Wiest

"Just five more minutes!" I used to tell myself while doing a cardio workout I absolutely hated. To me, cardio used to be the "gold standard" for exercise, and I never considered walks or doing yoga as a form of "real" movement even though I actually enjoyed doing them.

In a culture where many of us grew up with the saying of *"eat less and move more,"* oftentimes exercise is thought of as punishment for eating a brownie or the best way to lose weight. Fortunately, it doesn't have to be that way.

Maybe you can relate to my client who came to me struggling to lose weight despite eating only about twelve hundred calories and doing over an hour of cardio each day. She was doing everything she was taught by the book, yet her weight wasn't budging. I explained to her that over-restriction and too much cardio can actually prevent weight loss from happening. This is because it's a form of stress on the body and can contribute to a blood sugar roller-coaster disaster, ultimately preventing weight loss from happening.

Although I'm a true believer that you can't outrun a fork, exercise is an essential part of health—not just for the endorphins but also for the benefits it has on blood sugars and overall health.

HOW EXERCISE IMPACTS YOUR BLOOD SUGAR

Make a fist with your hand. Then open and close it five times.

You know what just happened? Your body used glucose to move your hand back and forth. That's because glucose is an important fuel for your muscles. When muscles contract during exercise, cells can use glucose for a quick burst of energy. Under normal conditions, over 80 percent of glucose uptake is from skeletal muscles. Not only does this help the body use up stored glucose, it also improves insulin sensitivity.

Along with the blood sugar benefits, exercise can reduce the risk for cardio-vascular disease and nerve damage, lower blood pressure, help you sleep better, improve memory, and support mental health. Feeling stressed? Exercise can help that too (Centers for Disease Control and Prevention 2022).

SHOULD I EAT BEFORE I EXERCISE?

The benefits on your blood sugar can change depending on whether you're fasting or non-fasting. A common question I get is, *"Should I eat before I exercise?"* My answer is generally yes, since it's a form of fuel for your workouts and can enhance performance during a workout. And for some people, working out without eating prior can dip blood glucose levels too low. On the flip side, there's some benefit to working-out fasted, like an increase in fat oxidation, which can lead to more fat loss. Ultimately, it depends on the time of your exercise, when your last meal or snack was, and the type of exercise you're doing. For example, you might not need to eat anything for a short walk in the morning, but it would be best to eat something prior to your morning spin class to give your body extra fuel for the more rigorous workout.

After exercise, I always recommend some type of meal or snack within thirty minutes that contains a source of complex carbohydrates and protein (like an apple and cottage cheese) to help repair and enhance muscle growth.

SIMPLE WAYS TO ADD MORE MOVEMENT TO YOUR DAY

Maybe exercise is something that gets put on the backburner when life gets busy. I get it. That's why I'm all about finding simple ways to add more movement to my day. Because let's be real—the average American is sedentary for over thirteen hours a day. Many of us are sitting in front of a computer working all day, then sitting more during our commute, then sitting once we get home. If you can get to the gym after work, great. If not, know that ten minutes here and there of what I call "exercise snacks" can add up quickly. If you did ten-minute exercise snacks three times a day, that would give you more than the recommended amount of exercise each week. Plus, even if you go to the gym or take a workout class, it's still important to sprinkle in activity throughout the entire day.

Here are some examples:

○ Use a stand-up desk at work or a walking treadmill.
○ Take a walk after a meal (one of the best times to move your body is after a meal for better blood sugar balance).
○ Do ten squats at the top of each hour during your workday.
○ March in place or walk around while talking on the phone.
○ Do a ten-minute strength training workout on YouTube.
○ Perform yoga stretches first thing in the morning and before bed.
○ Take the stairs whenever possible.
○ Park far away in a parking lot.
○ Do ten-minute breaks with push-ups, jumping jacks, and lunges.

THE BENEFITS OF STRENGTH TRAINING

Along with movements like biking or walking, one of the most beneficial workouts you can do is some form of strength training. Not only is it great for building muscle and enhancing glucose metabolism, it also helps keep bones strong, reduces the risk for cardiovascular disease, and can help reduce joint pain. One meta-analysis study found that those who did a form of strength training for just thirty to sixty minutes a week also had a 10 to 20 percent lower mortality risk (Momma et al. 2022).

Current US exercise guidelines recommend adults do a form of strength training for all major muscle groups at least twice per week. This can be in the form of weightlifting or exercises like push-ups, lunges, or sit-ups (Centers for Disease Control and Prevention 2022).

GETTING INTO A CONSISTENT WORKOUT ROUTINE

Now that you know that doing burpees until you're red in the face does not need to be the gold standard for exercise, what should you do for exercise? It's important to get all the benefits of exercise without it being too stressful on the body. Here's an example of a workout routine that can be a great place to start no matter what your health goals are.

1. Start with consistent walks or other lower-intensity workouts like yoga, Pilates, swimming, or biking.

2. Add in strength training two to four times per week.

3. Sprinkle in high-intensity workouts or longer-duration cardio if your nutrition, sleep, and stress are well managed.

There might be days when you're totally game for a spin class and other days when all you want to do is lie in the dark in a restorative yoga class. If you have a menstrual cycle, know that hormonal changes throughout your cycle can influence your desire and energy for exercise. For example, the follicular phase (first part of the cycle) is often the best time for more strength training or higher-intensity workouts. The luteal phase (the second part of your cycle) is a time when you may be more inclined to do less-intense workouts.

Ultimately, what's most important is finding an exercise routine you *actually* enjoy and can fit into your schedule. Because an exercise routine that's enjoyable and easy to implement is a lot more sustainable.

REFLECTION

1. What are exercises you enjoy doing? What are some ways you can make exercise more fun?

----

2. What are one to three "exercise snacks" you could incorporate into your day?

CHAPTER 17

THE IMPORTANCE OF ZZZ'S FOR BALANCED BLOOD SUGARS

"True power is living the realization that you are your own healer, hero, and leader."

—Yung Pueblo

Insomnia and sleep issues are pervasive in our culture. In fact, about one-third of adults are sleep deprived (meaning they report getting less than seven hours of sleep each night). With higher levels of stress, and exposure to electronics everywhere, it's no wonder so many of us are yawning all day. The importance of sleep is often overlooked, despite it playing a significant role in many aspects of health, including blood sugar regulation, improving moods, supporting hormone production, and assisting in nervous system function.

WHAT HAPPENS IF I DON'T GET ENOUGH SLEEP?

You've probably felt tired after a night of not-so-great sleep, but what else happens if you don't get enough sleep?

We often sacrifice sleep due to busy work schedules, stress, family obligations, social media, or that binge-worthy show on Netflix. Unfortunately, many of us are not realizing the hormonal imbalances and stress on the body this is causing.

For optimal health, it's recommended to get at least seven to nine hours of quality sleep each night. Sleep from the hours of ten p.m. to six a.m. aligns well with your body's natural production of melatonin, the hormone regulating your sleep-wake cycle.

Sometimes people rely on "catching up" on sleep on the weekends. Although you can do this to a certain extent, it's pretty challenging to make up all the sleep debt you owe. For example, if you sleep six hours a night during the week, you'll need to sleep an extra five hours (at minimum) on the weekend.

Sleep is the foundational time for the body to heal, detox, and repair. Every system and hormone is getting recharged during this time, including our appetite hormones. Have you felt more hungry or had more sugar cravings after a night of not-so-great sleep? You can blame your appetite hormones for that one.

Ghrelin, the "hunger hormone" that secretes when your stomach is empty and it's time to eat, increases with a lack of sleep, while leptin, the "fullness hormone" that helps prevent hunger and regulates energy balance, will fall without adequate sleep. This means that a lack of sleep directly impacts your energy balance and hunger the next day by increasing the "I'm hungry" hormone and decreasing your "I'm full" hormone.

Along with the appetite hormones, cortisol can be elevated without enough sleep. With this increase in cortisol, the release of other hormones (such as melatonin) are negatively impacted. Let's not also forget the health complications of a lack of "zzz's," like an increased risk for heart disease, depression, obesity, type 2 diabetes, and certain cancers. It's also linked to a higher risk for injuries and cognitive decline (National Heart, Lung, and Blood Institute 2022).

Maybe you already know the importance of sleep, but you work the night shift or have kids waking you up during the night. If that's the case, it's important to focus on what you can control—your *quality* of sleep and sleep routine.

IMPROVING YOUR SLEEP ROUTINE

The older I get, the more important my sleep routine becomes, and if you know you need to improve your sleep but you're not sure exactly how, here are some things to try.

Get morning sunlight: Why am I talking about the morning when we're talking about bedtime? Because what you do in the morning can influence your circadian rhythm, and getting morning sunlight plays a crucial role in regulating the sleep-wake cycle. This one change can have a positive impact on your late-night "zzz's" by resetting your biological clock. Try getting outside right after waking up to get some sunlight on your face (without sunglasses), or use a sun lamp to help improve your sleep (and improve mood).

Avoid eating right before bed: I'm all about a bedtime snack if you need one, but eating too close to bedtime can be disruptive. That's because a late bedtime snack causes your body to focus on digestion versus resting. So if you're having an evening snack, try to have it more than an hour before bedtime.

Try adding magnesium: Since magnesium is a muscle relaxant, it can be a great supplement to take an hour before bed to help prepare it for bedtime. I've heard countless times, and have also experienced, the positive impact magnesium can have on sleep quality. Two hundred to four hundred milligrams of a magnesium glycinate supplement can be a great place to start. *As with any supplement, it's important to check the quality, and work with your healthcare provider before trying something new.*

Limit electronics one to two hours before bed: I know, I know. What about the late-night show you're binge watching or the hour after the kids go to bed where you can catch up on social media? This is often the hardest one for most people. But the blue light emitted from electronics prevents the production of melatonin, making it hard to fall asleep or get restful sleep. It's best to limit electronics, including television, phone, computers, tablets, etc. for one to two hours before light's out. If that's not possible, invest in some high-quality blue-light-blocking glasses to help prevent exposure.

Avoid alcohol before bed: While a late-night glass of wine may make you feel sleepy, it's not so great for your sleep quality. That's because when the liver enzymes are metabolizing alcohol, it can disrupt your natural sleep cycle. It can also cause sleep apnea or sleep disorders to worsen (Sleep Foundation 2024).

Assess your bedroom: Is your bedroom environment set up for a calming sleep routine? According to the Sleep Foundation, it's best to sleep in a cooler environment, around 65 degrees Fahrenheit. It may be no surprise that a quieter environment makes it easier to sleep better. If that's not possible, using a white-noise machine can be helpful for blocking out disruptive sounds. Lastly, when it comes to light, hues of red, orange, and yellow make it easier for the body to prepare for sleep versus blue light (like from your electronics mentioned above), which makes it more difficult. Lastly, consider putting your cell phone on silent (or better yet, not even in your bedroom) to prevent distractions, and try some drops of lavender essential oils on your pillow to help promote relaxation (Sleep Foundation 2024).

WHAT IF I CAN FALL ASLEEP FINE, BUT I CAN'T STAY ASLEEP?

So what if you can fall asleep like a champ but can never actually stay asleep at night? There could be an underlying reason for this, like one of these.

Stress: If you're under a lot of stress, cortisol is working overtime, and it's blocking the regular rhythm of melatonin. Finding something to help relax and calm the mind before bed can be a good start. Try doing a ten-minute guided meditation or breathing exercise or listening to calming music while stretching. If you feel like your mind is all over the place before bed, try keeping a journal on your nightstand and write down any thoughts or ideas that come up.

Low blood sugars: If you tend to wake up during the night, especially around three in the morning, this can be a sign of low blood sugars. Since we're not eating while we're sleeping, the body gradually raises cortisol to help stimulate the body to release or create enough glucose to supply the brain with energy. Those with chronic low blood sugars, however, tend to have difficulty making the right amount of cortisol to help fuel the brain with enough glucose. If this is you, I recommend adding in a bedtime snack with complex carbohydrates and some protein/fat. For example, you could try sprouted toast with almond butter or berries with coconut cream.

Certain medications: Some medications can influence sleep and cause wakings in the middle of the night. Those can include beta-blockers, diuretics, and antidepressants (Sleep Foundation 2014).

Prioritizing sleep each night can improve your energy, stress levels, cardiovascular and mental health, and blood sugars. Here's to a good night's sleep tonight and every night!

REFLECTION

1. *Now that you know how important sleep is for overall health, how can you improve your sleep routine? Maybe that means replacing that evening wine for some chamomile tea, and the late-night TV show for some reading. Write some ideas below.*

CHAPTER 18

ARE THERE SUPPLEMENTS TO HELP IMPROVE BLOOD SUGAR?

"Who you are tomorrow begins with what you do today."

—Tim Fargo

While I'm all about food first, there are several supplements that can give your body extra blood sugar support. We've talked about some to help with digestion and stress, but what about blood sugar management, specifically? Here are some helpful ones.

Berberine: This compound extracted from plants has a long history in Chinese medicine for its various health benefits. It's thought to work by activating an enzyme inside the cells called AMP-activated protein kinase, which plays a role in metabolism and energy (Jin et al. 2017). A review of twenty-seven studies found taking berberine in combination with diet and lifestyle changes reduced fasting glucose and hemoglobin A1C compared to the placebo (Lan et al. 2015). Other studies have found berberine to reduce insulin resistance and the uptake of insulin in those with type 2 diabetes (Cao and Su 2019).
Dosage: 500 mg three times per day

Magnesium glycinate: Magnesium has been shown to reduce fasting plasma glucose in individuals with diabetes and those at risk for diabetes. More recent studies have found higher levels of magnesium to be associated with an increase in insulin sensitivity (Dastgerdi et al. 2022). Bonus—it can provide a calming effect on the body, which can also support blood sugar levels.

Dosage: 200–400 mg per day

Vitamin D: This nutrient has been shown to improve insulin sensitivity and help regulate glucose levels by stimulating the release of insulin from the pancreas. One study found a significant difference in glycemic control in those with type 1 diabetes after supplementing with vitamin D for twelve weeks (Aljabri et al. 2010). Along with that, vitamin D can be helpful for improving moods and supporting bone health. Getting your vitamin D level checked annually is something I often recommend, especially if you live in an environment that doesn't have sunlight all year long.

Dosage: can vary depending on the time of year and your serum 25(OH) D levels. An optimal range for vitamin D is between 50–80 ng/mL. If you're below that level, consider supplementation. A general dosage is between 2,000–5,000 IU per day.

Omega-3 fatty acids: These heart-healthy fats are not only great for reducing stress and inflammation in the body, they've also been found to improve insulin sensitivity (Lepretti et al. 2018).

Dosage: 1,000–2,000 mg per day with meals

Alpha lipoic acid (ALA): This is a powerful antioxidant that is often recommended for those with metabolic syndrome, PCOS, and obesity. It's been found to help lower blood sugar levels by increasing glucose uptake into cells (Capece et al. 2022).

Dosage: 100 mg three times daily before each meal

Remember, always work with your healthcare provider before trying a new supplement.

OTHER TOOLS TO SUPPORT BLOOD SUGAR REGULATION

Along with supplementation, certain spices can also be used as a supplement to enhance blood sugars at meals. They include:

○ **Cinnamon:** This can be added to coffee, tea, oatmeal, or smoothies (aim for at least ½ to 1 teaspoon daily).

○ **Fenugreek:** This can be added to soups, rice, or marinades.

○ **Turmeric:** Use in egg bakes or in the golden milk recipe in the back of the book. Be sure to use it with black pepper to enhance absorption.

○ **Ginger:** Add this to teas or stir fries.

> **Quick tip:** Along with prioritizing balanced meals and snacks, adding certain supplements, such as magnesium or berberine, can help provide additional support for optimal blood sugar levels.

CHAPTER 19

PUTTING IT ALL TOGETHER

"A slight change in your daily habits can guide your life to a very different destination."

—James Clear

Maybe this is the point where you have so many great ideas and feel inspired to take action, yet you don't really know where to begin.

This chapter is all about breaking it down for you.

Maybe you've tried a diet or health program before and made several changes during the program, but once you went back to your normal way of living, you were back to ground zero. This is common, and often a result of not learning *behavior changes.* Sure, many of us could follow an "eat this" list or workout plan for a couple of weeks, but once we don't have someone telling us exactly what to do all the time, we fall off track.

One thing I often recommend to clients is to look at your health like a marathon versus a 100-meter sprint. With the popularity of Amazon Prime and same-day Target pickup, we get used to these quick and instant results. Our health is not like that though. Blood sugar issues, excess belly fat, sugar cravings, brain fog, or constant fatigue didn't just show up overnight, so they're not going to disappear overnight either.

You probably have routines around hundreds of daily things, like how you drive to the grocery store, how you brush your teeth, or the first thing you do when you get to work. These are all routines you had to learn. You weren't just born with the natural ability to tie your shoe, were you?

And that's the same with any new health endeavor. It must be implemented and learned so it becomes a habit too.

HOW TO MAKE CHANGES THAT LAST

Something I always encourage clients to do is focus on one to three action items at a time. Many people want to go all in and see the greatest impact in a short amount of time. They might change fifteen different things at once, then get burnt out, and end up not making any changes at all. This doesn't have to be the case for you. Here are some ideas on how to make changes that last.

Make super specific action goals: When I say super specific, I mean *super* specific. Instead of goals like, "I'm going to eat more vegetables," try breaking it down and be as detailed as possible. For example, "I'm going to eat one cup of vegetables at lunch and dinner three days per week." This is a much more specific goal that tells you what you're going to do, when you're going to do it, and how often. The more specific a goal is, the easier it will be to achieve it.

Add auditory or visual cues: A simple auditory or visual cue can be a game-changer for helping you remember to do an action item. For example, put a Post-it note on your fridge to help you remember to pack an afternoon snack for work, a timer on your phone to remind you to take a stretch break, or place a couple of filled water bottles on your counter so you remember to drink them.

Stack your habits: Habit stacking is a topic that James Clear talks a lot about in his book *Atomic Habits*, which means to build new habits around old ones. This makes building new healthier habits into your day easier because it doesn't require adding a lot more on your to-do list.

The habit stacking formula is: After/Before [CURRENT HABIT], I will [NEW HABIT].

Here are some examples:

- After I brew my morning coffee, I will drink one cup of water.
- Before I turn on the shower, I will think of five things I'm grateful for.
- After I eat lunch, I will go for a ten-minute walk.
- Before I lie in my bed, I will put my phone on airplane mode.

Set up your environment for success: Prior to becoming a registered dietitian, I worked in corporate wellness where I would help businesses create a healthier environment for their employees. Things like vending machine options or types of breakroom snacks were easy common changes, and you can use this same concept at home. When you look around your home (especially your kitchen) does it promote health? Do you have vegetables and fruit readily available to grab in your fridge? Or do you have chocolate chip cookies in your cupboard that you constantly have to restrain yourself from? Keeping nourishing foods more obvious and easier to grab will make eating more nourishing foods a whole lot easier.

Focus on sustainability: I love all the clients who are really ambitious and tell me they're going to implement a new change seven days a week. Although some people are rock stars like that, more often than not, it's not very realistic or sustainable for most people. It takes time to build a new habit, so it's important to give yourself some grace if it's not perfect at first. Maybe three workouts a week is more sustainable than five workouts right now. Maybe making dinners at home five days a week is more realistic than making dinner all week long. Think about what's sustainable and realistic for you.

CELEBRATE YOUR WINS

Every week I encourage clients to celebrate their wins, whether big or small. It's easy to only celebrate once you hit your big ultimate goal, but what about the small milestones along the way? Those often get brushed off, but those are the most important times to celebrate. For example, if you have a goal to lose twenty pounds, I'd encourage you to celebrate every time you lose another five pounds. Those small milestone celebrations will give you the encouragement to continue on the journey.

Many times we celebrate with food, like ice cream or chocolate. Instead, I encourage you to find non-food-related ways to celebrate your wins. Things like buying yourself a new book or flowers, going for a hike at a new place, or sleeping in on Saturday morning are some ideas.

GET BACK ON THE WAGON

Improving your health isn't going to be all rainbows and sunshine. There are going to be times when you might slip up or fall off the wagon. What's most important is that you focus on getting back on, and don't let one not-so-great day turn into two, four, or a week. In the words of James Clear, *"Never miss twice."*

> **Quick tip:** The more specific a goal is, the easier it is to accomplish. When setting any new health goal, make sure it's SMART (specific, measurable, achievable, relevant, and time-bound).

REFLECTION

1. *Think about where you want to be one year from now. What are some of your current habits that are supportive of where you want to be in a year? How can you do those more often?*

2. *Next, what are some of your current habits that aren't supportive of where you want to be in a year? How can you eliminate or reduce those?*

----

3. *Lastly, what are one to three small, specific action items to start doing in the next few days to get you closer to your health goals based on the information you've learned so far? Remember, the more specific, the easier to accomplish!*

FINAL THOUGHTS

You made it! We've covered a lot in this book, and you now have a variety of tricks, tools, and knowledge to support your blood sugars and overall health.

My hope is that you realize how truly powerful you are in changing the quality of your health. Wellness isn't a state of mind; it's a state of action. You just have to get started.

I know many people want a magic pill to take their health problems away, but there isn't one. Your health is a journey, and one single food, medication, or specific habit can't magically fix all your health problems. Supporting your blood sugars with balanced, nutrient-dense foods is the number-one foundational piece of good health, and you now have several tools and strategies to do just that.

Although some of these new changes may seem daunting right now or something you constantly have to think about, know that it will get easier. Eventually following PFF at your meals, adding minerals to your water, or always pairing a carb with a buddy will become automatic and something that comes naturally like brushing your teeth.

If you're looking for additional support, be sure to find me on Instagram and Facebook @autumn.enloe.nutrition and my website: https://autumnenloe.com.

And grab your free resources, including printable macronutrient and glycemic index guides, a grocery shopping list, and my favorite supplement brands (and more!) to further assist you with the contents of this book at https://autumnenloe.com/bloodsugarbook.

Last but not least, if you could take two minutes to leave a review of this book on whatever platform you found it, to help others learn about the power of nutrition and how blood sugar regulation is such a foundational piece of health as you've learned, I will be forever grateful.

In the next section you'll find over forty delicious, simple, and balanced recipes that I know you'll love. They're packed with nutrients like protein and vegetables to support balanced blood sugars all day long. You'll also find a sample meal plan using the 1-2-3 meal-prepping method to help you utilize these recipes.

Remember, you only have one body to live in. Nourish it well.

I'm cheering you on.

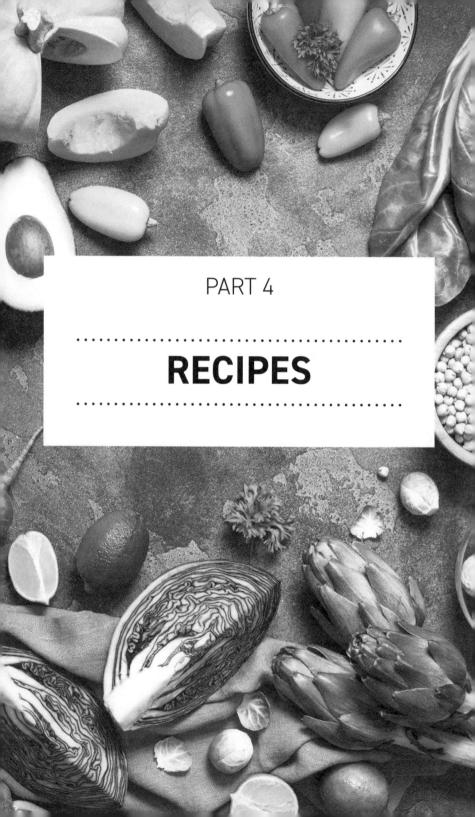

PART 4

....

RECIPES

....

SAMPLE MEAL PLAN

This sample meal plan uses the 1-2-3 method described in Chapter 13. Feel free to adjust, depending on your needs. The 1-2-3 method includes one main option for breakfast, alternating between two options for lunch, and alternating between three options, including leftovers, for dinner.

	Week 1	Week 2	Week 3	Week 4
Breakfast	Banana Bread Oatmeal Bake (page 126)	Cheesy Broccoli Egg Bake + Side of Fruit (page 128)	Tropical Green Smoothie (page 132)	PB and J Yogurt Bowl (page 130)
Lunch	Italian Vegetable Soup (page 135) + Fruit Cucumber, Tomato, and Feta Salad (page 141) + Chicken	Dill and Cucumber Chicken Salad (page 141) Thai Crunch Salad (page 144) + Turkey	Lemon Pepper Salmon Salad (page 143) Served in a Wrap + Veggies Easy Egg Salad (page 142) + Veggies	Strawberry Goat Cheese Salad (page 143) + Chicken Beef and Veggie Chili (page 133)
Dinner	Broccoli and Beef Rice Bowls (page 133) Sheet-Pan Chicken Curry (page 137) Turkey Taco Casserole (page 139)	Mediterranean Meatballs and Veggies (page 136) Veggie Spaghetti Bake (page 140) Beef and Veggie Chili (page 133)	Shrimp and Cabbage Bowls (page 138) Parmesan Chicken and Veggies (page 137) Italian Vegetable Soup (page 135) + Side Salad	Turkey Taco Casserole (page 139) Broccoli and Beef Rice Bowls (page 133) Crockpot Chicken Tortilla Soup (page 134)
Snacks Options	Everything But the Bagel Veggie Dip (page 147) With Veggies + Hard-Boiled Egg Almond Butter Bars (page 145)	Yogurt Fruit Dip (page 149) + Strawberries Chocolate Chia Seed Pudding (page 146)	Chocolate Chip Peanut Butter Bars (page 147) Tuna Cucumber Bites (page 149)	Apple Cinnamon Cottage Cheese (page 145) Trail Mix Peanut Butter Balls (page 148)

BREAKFAST

Banana Bread Oatmeal Bake

This is a flavor-packed oatmeal bake for your busy mornings! Prep this on the weekend, and heat it up in minutes for a quick breakfast all week long.

Serves: 8 | **Prep/Cook Time:** 30 minutes

2 cups oats
4 scoops unflavored collagen powder
½ tablespoon cinnamon
½ teaspoon baking soda
¼ teaspoon nutmeg
¼ teaspoon sea salt

1 cup mashed banana (about 2 to 3 medium bananas)
4 eggs
¼ cup maple syrup
1 teaspoon vanilla extract

1. Preheat the oven to 375°F and grease an 8×8-inch pan with nonstick spray. You could also cut a piece of parchment paper and place it at the bottom of the pan as a liner.

2. In a small bowl, combine the oats, collagen, cinnamon, baking soda, nutmeg, and salt. Stir well.

3. In a large bowl, mash the bananas until they're completely soft.

4. Whisk in the eggs, then stir in the maple syrup and vanilla.

5. Add the oat mixture to the wet ingredients and stir to combine them.

6. Pour the mixture into a baking dish and bake for 25 minutes or until golden brown.

7. To serve: heat up and mix in your milk of choice. I also love to top it off with some banana slices and walnuts.

> (Per 1 slice) **Calories:** 279, **Protein:** 25 grams,
> **Carbohydrates:** 30 grams, **Fat:** 8 grams

Breakfast Veggie Scramble

This is an easy way to get vegetables and protein from the very beginning of the day. You can switch up the vegetables based on what you have on hand. Serve it with fruit on the side.

Serves: 2 | **Prep/Cook Time:** 15 minutes

1 teaspoon avocado oil

1 cup broccoli, chopped into small pieces

4 nitrate-free breakfast sausages, diced

1 cup chopped kale

5 eggs, beaten

1 teaspoon Italian seasoning

⅛ teaspoon black pepper

⅛ teaspoon sea salt

Toppings: parsley, avocado slices, feta cheese (optional)

1. Heat the avocado oil in a pan over medium heat.

2. Add in the broccoli and nitrate-free breakfast sausages, and sauté them for 5 minutes.

3. Add the kale and continue to cook it until it's wilted.

4. Meanwhile, mix the eggs and spices together in a bowl. Add the mixture to the pan.

5. Continue to cook everything until the eggs are cooked through.

6. Add some toppings, if desired, and serve.

Note: Look for breakfast sausages that don't contain sodium nitrates, which are a harmful preservative found in some processed meats.

Calories: 421, **Protein:** 30 grams, **Carbohydrates:** 12 grams, **Fat:** 28 grams

Cinnamon Nut Granola

This easy homemade granola is a delicious topping for any yogurt! Made with simple ingredients, you'll never want to buy store-bought granola again.

Makes: 6 cups | **Prep/Cook Time:** 40 minutes

4 cups oats

1 cup slivered almonds

1 cup chopped pecans

½ cup coconut oil, melted

½ cup honey or maple syrup

2 tablespoons cinnamon

1 teaspoon vanilla extract

½ teaspoon sea salt

1. Preheat the oven to 350°F.

2. Line a large-rimmed baking sheet with parchment paper and set it aside.

3. In a large mixing bowl, combine all the ingredients. Mix them well until everything is well coated.

4. Spread the granola mixture on the baking sheet.

5. Bake the mixture in the oven for 25–30 minutes, or until it's golden brown. Stir the mixture halfway through.

6. Remove the mixture from the oven, and allow it to cool undistributed for about 30 minutes. The granola will crisp up as it cools.

7. Store in the refrigerator, or freeze extras for later.

> **(Per ½ cup) Calories:** 270, **Protein:** 5 grams,
> **Carbohydrates:** 30 grams, **Fat:** 15 grams

Cheesy Broccoli Egg Bake

This tasty and high-protein egg bake is a mix of greens and cheese, which make a perfect combo for any breakfast! I love adding turmeric to egg bakes to get in some extra antioxidants. Pair it with some fruit or sourdough for a complete breakfast.

Makes: 6 slices | **Prep/Cook Time:** 55 minutes

2½ cups chopped broccoli
½ cup minced green onions
(about 3 total)
12 eggs
1 cup shredded cheese
½ cup cottage cheese

1 teaspoon garlic powder
½ teaspoon turmeric
¼ teaspoon sea salt
¼ teaspoon black pepper

1. Preheat the oven to 375°F.

2. Spray a 9x9-inch baking pan with cooking spray.

3. Spread the chopped broccoli and green onions on the bottom of the baking dish.

4. In a large mixing bowl, combine the remaining ingredients.

5. Pour the mixture on top of the broccoli and green onions.

6. Bake the mixture in the oven for 45 minutes, or until a toothpick inserted into the middle of the egg bake comes out clean.

> (Per 1 slice) **Calories:** 236, **Protein:** 20 grams,
> **Carbohydrates:** 5 grams, **Fat:** 16 grams

Chocolate Banana Smoothie

Have your chocolate without all the sugar! Packed with protein, this smoothie is a great way to get in a variety of nutrients from the very beginning of your day.

Serves: 1 | **Prep/Cook Time:** 5 minutes

1 serving of chocolate protein powder (at least 20 grams of protein)

1 small banana

1 cup spinach

1 tablespoon natural peanut butter

½ cup milk or water for blending

3 to 4 ice cubes

1. Add all the ingredients in the blender, and blend them until they're smooth.

> **Calories:** 422, **Protein:** 26 grams, **Carbohydrates:** 38 grams, **Fat:** 20 grams

Mediterranean Veggie Egg Cups

These easy egg cups are packed with veggies and flavor! Simply heat them up for a quick option for breakfast. Pair them with a fibrous carbohydrate to complete the meal.

Makes: 12 egg cups | **Prep/Cook Time:** 35 minutes

1 cup spinach, diced

½ cup red bell pepper, diced

⅓ cup feta cheese

12 eggs

1 teaspoon garlic powder

1 teaspoon Italian seasoning

⅛ teaspoon black pepper

⅛ teaspoon sea salt

1. Preheat the oven to 350°F.

2. Spray a 12-cup muffin pan with nonstick spray or use muffin liners.

3. Place the spinach and peppers into each muffin tin. Top with feta cheese (*can omit if dairy-free*).

4. In a medium bowl, mix the eggs with all the spices.

5. Pour the egg mixture into each individual muffin tin until it's about ¾ filled.

6. Bake egg mixture in the oven for 25 minutes, or until a toothpick inserted into the middle comes out clean.

> **(For 2 egg cups) Calories:** 309, **Protein:** 26 grams, **Carbohydrates:** 4 grams, **Fat:** 21 grams

PB and J Yogurt Bowl

A combination of sweet and savory, this PB and J Yogurt bowl is simple to make, and is a filling breakfast that will support stable blood sugars all morning long. Make several servings of this at once for an easy breakfast on the go!

Makes: 1 cup | **Prep/Cook Time:** 5 minutes

1 cup plain Greek yogurt

1 tablespoon Mixed Berry Chia Jam

1 tablespoon natural peanut butter

¼ cup diced strawberries

1 tablespoon nuts of choice (such as walnuts, pecans, or slivered almonds)

1. Place the plain Greek yogurt in a bowl.

2. Add the chia jam, peanut butter, strawberries, and nuts on top.

Mixed Berry Chia Jam

Makes: 1 cup | **Prep/Cook Time:** 30 minutes

2 cups frozen mixed berries

1 tablespoon maple syrup

2 tablespoons chia seeds

1. Add the mixed berries to a small pot and heat them on medium heat. Bring the berries to a boil for 5 minutes.

2. Reduce the heat to simmer, and cover the berries for 5 minutes.

3. Remove the berries from the heat, and mash them with a fork or potato masher.

4. Stir in the maple syrup and chia seeds.

5. Let the berries cool for 20 minutes (the jam will thicken over time).

6. Store the jam in an airtight container in the refrigerator for up to 7 days.

> **Calories:** 317, **Protein:** 25 grams, **Carbohydrates:** 26 grams, **Fat:** 13 grams

Protein Pancakes

This is a classic breakfast meal with a twist! Don't let the cottage cheese scare you—it adds more protein and helps create fluffy pancakes that will keep you coming back for more. Top them with natural nut butter, berries, or a little maple syrup for a balanced breakfast.

Makes: about 10 (4-inch) pancakes | **Prep/Cook Time:** 15 minutes

1½ cups cottage cheese	2 teaspoons cinnamon
4 eggs	1 teaspoon baking powder
2 cups almond flour	2 tablespoons coconut oil, divided
2 teaspoons vanilla extract	

1. Mix all the ingredients (except the coconut oil) in a mixing bowl until they're well combined.

2. Heat a large skillet over medium heat. Add ½ tablespoon of coconut oil to the skillet.

3. Using an ice cream scooper, add the batter to the skillet to make each individual pancake.

4. Once little bubbles form in the batter, flip the pancakes and cook them until they're golden.

5. Continue adding coconut oil to the pan, and repeat steps 2–4 until all the batter is gone.

> **(Per 1 pancake) Calories:** 115, **Protein:** 8 grams,
> **Carbohydrates:** 3 grams, **Fat:** 8 grams

Strawberry Overnight Oats

Here's an easy breakfast option that's full of fiber and protein that will keep you feeling full for hours. You can easily prep a couple of servings at once to have breakfast ready for days!

Serves: 1 | **Prep/Cook Time:** 5 minutes

1 cup plain Greek yogurt
½ cup chopped strawberries
½ cup rolled oats
¼ cup milk of choice

1 tablespoon chia seeds
1 teaspoon honey
½ teaspoon vanilla extract

1. Add all the ingredients to a 16-ounce mason jar or other similar container.

2. Mix well until the ingredients are well combined.

3. Store covered overnight in the refrigerator.

4. Serve cold and top with more strawberries if desired.

Calories: 304, **Protein:** 25 grams, **Carbohydrates:** 38 grams, **Fat:** 7 grams

Tropical Green Smoothie

A refreshing smoothie packed with green vegetables that makes a balanced breakfast to start your day!

Serves: 1 | **Prep/Cook Time:** 5 minutes

1 serving of vanilla protein powder
(at least 20 grams of protein)
1 cup spinach
1 cup frozen pineapple

½ cup diced zucchini
½ cup milk or water for blending
½ teaspoon vanilla extract

1. Add all the ingredients to the blender, and blend them until they're smooth.

Calories: 335, **Protein:** 20 grams, **Carbohydrates:** 30 grams, **Fat:** 4 grams

MAIN DISHES

Beef and Veggie Chili

This is a veggie-packed chili you'll love! This comforting dish can be made in the Crockpot and tastes even better as leftovers.

Serves: 6 | **Prep/Cook Time:** 4–6 hours

1 pound lean ground beef (opt for grass-fed if you can)

1 onion, diced

1 cup diced carrots

1 bell pepper, diced (any color)

2 (15-ounce) cans kidney beans, rinsed and drained

1 (28-ounce) can crushed tomatoes

1 cup vegetable or beef broth

1 tablespoon dijon mustard

½ tablespoon ground cumin

½ teaspoon paprika

½ teaspoon chili powder

⅛ teaspoon sea salt

⅛ teaspoon black pepper

Toppings: fresh cilantro, avocado, plain Greek yogurt, or cheese (optional)

1. In a medium pan, cook the meat until it's no longer pink. Add the chopped onion, carrots, and peppers, and sauté for 5 minutes. Once done, add them to a large Crockpot.

2. Add all the remaining ingredients to a Crockpot and cook on low for 6 hours, or on high for 4 hours.

3. Add toppings if desired.

Calories: 353, **Protein:** 26 grams, **Carbohydrates:** 59 grams, **Fat:** 4 grams

Broccoli and Beef Rice Bowls

This easy dish tastes better than take-out and can be made in just 30 minutes! I love to make this in my cast-iron pan, so if you do that, you can omit the avocado oil.

Serves: 4 | **Prep/Cook Time:** 30 minutes

2 cups cooked brown rice

1 tablespoon avocado oil

1 pound ribeye steak, cut into strips

4 cups chopped broccoli

2 cups diced carrots
1 onion, diced
½ cup coconut aminos (an alternative to soy sauce)
2 tablespoons rice vinegar
1 tablespoon minced garlic
¼ teaspoon black pepper
¼ teaspoon sea salt
Toppings: red pepper flakes, sesame seeds, or green onions (optional)

1. Cook the rice according to its package directions.

2. In a large pan, add the avocado oil on medium heat. Add the strips of steak.

3. Add the broccoli, carrots, and onions, and cook them until the steak is no longer pink and the vegetables are tender.

4. Meanwhile, combine the coconut aminos, rice vinegar, garlic, black pepper, and salt in a bowl. Mix well.

5. Pour the sauce over the steak with vegetables. Mix well, and cook for an additional 1 to 2 minutes.

6. Serve over cooked rice, and add toppings if desired.

Calories: 364, **Protein:** 31 grams, **Carbohydrates:** 43 grams, **Fat:** 7 grams

Crockpot Chicken Tortilla Soup

Here's a delicious veggie and protein-packed soup! Simply mix all the ingredients together, and leave it in the Crockpot for later.

Serves: 4–5 | **Prep/Cook Time:** 6–8 hours

1½ pounds raw chicken breast
32 ounces chicken broth
1 (15-ounce) can black beans, rinsed and drained
10 ounces frozen corn
1 cup salsa
4 Roma tomatoes, diced
1 bell pepper, diced
½ tablespoon ground cumin
½ tablespoon garlic powder
¼ teaspoon paprika
⅛ teaspoon sea salt
⅛ teaspoon black pepper
Toppings: cilantro, tortilla chips, avocado slices, plain Greek yogurt, or shredded cheese (optional)

1. Place all the ingredients into a large Crockpot and mix well. Cook on low heat for 8 hours or on high heat for 6 hours.

2. Once done, remove the chicken breast, and cut it into small pieces (make sure the chicken is at least 165°F before serving).

3. Add toppings if desired.

Calories: 310, **Protein:** 24 grams, **Carbohydrates:** 44 grams, **Fat:** 7 grams

Italian Vegetable Soup

This is one of my favorite soups for cooler months. This comforting veggie-packed soup can be made in just 30 minutes. Double the batch, and freeze the extras for later!

Serves: 4 | **Prep/Cook Time:** 30 minutes

1 pound ground pork

1 onion, diced

2 cups diced carrots

3 celery sticks, diced

2 cups diced baby potatoes

6 cups vegetable broth

½ tablespoon Italian seasoning

1 teaspoon garlic powder

¼ teaspoon black pepper

¼ teaspoon sea salt

2 cups chopped kale

1. In a large soup pot, brown the ground pork on medium heat until it's no longer pink. Transfer the ground pork to a bowl, and set it aside.

2. Add the onions, carrots, and celery into the soup pot and sauté them for 5 to 7 minutes, or until the onions are translucent.

3. Add the potatoes, broth, seasonings, and pork into the pot. Mix well.

4. Increase the heat, and bring the soup to a boil.

6. Reduce the heat to simmer. Cover the soup, and continue to cook it for 20 minutes.

7. Once the time is up, remove the cover and add the chopped kale.

8. Continue to cook the soup on simmer until the kale is wilted—about 5 minutes.

9. Allow the soup to cool for 10 minutes before serving it.

Calories: 353, **Protein:** 28 grams, **Carbohydrates:** 24 grams, **Fat:** 17 grams

Mediterranean Turkey Meatballs and Veggies

This is a Mediterranean-inspired dish composed of several different vegetables, chickpeas, and meatballs. Make a double batch to use for a simple lunch or dinner throughout the week!

Serves: 4 | **Prep/Cook Time:** 35 minutes

Vegetables and Chickpeas

1 (15-ounce) can chickpeas, rinsed and drained

2 bell peppers, cut into strips

1 onion, cut into strips

1 zucchini, cut into strips

1 tablespoon avocado oil

1 teaspoon garlic powder

1 teaspoon oregano

½ teaspoon black pepper

½ teaspoon sea salt

Meatballs

1 pound ground turkey

2 tablespoons almond flour

1 egg, beaten

1 teaspoon Italian seasoning

1 teaspoon garlic powder

½ cup feta cheese

1. Preheat the oven to 400°F. Line two large baking pans with parchment paper.

2. In a large bowl, mix together all the ingredients for the vegetable and chickpea mixture.

3. Pour the vegetables and chickpeas onto one of the baking pans, and roast them in the oven for 10 minutes.

4. While the vegetables are cooking, make the meatballs by mixing all the ingredients together in a bowl. Shape the meatballs into 1-inch balls and place them on the other baking pan. *Omit the cheese if dairy-free.*

5. Once 10 minutes are up for the vegetables, remove them from oven and flip them over.

6. Place the pan with the vegetables back in the oven along with the pan of meatballs and cook them for 20 minutes or until the meatballs reach 165°F.

7. Serve the meatballs over the vegetable mixture.

Calories: 413, **Protein:** 30 grams, **Carbohydrates:** 30 grams, **Fat:** 20 grams

Parmesan Garlic Chicken and Veggies

This one-pan dish is a great balance of all the macronutrients. It's simple, flavorful, and done in just 30 minutes!

Serves: 4 | **Prep/Cook Time:** 30 minutes

1½ pounds chicken breast, diced into 1-inch pieces
6 cups diced broccoli
6 cups diced cauliflower
3 tablespoons avocado oil

1 tablespoon garlic powder
½ teaspoon black pepper
½ teaspoon sea salt
½ cup parmesan cheese, plus additional for topping

1. Preheat the oven to 450°F. Line a large baking pan with parchment paper.

2. In a large bowl, coat the chicken, broccoli, and cauliflower with the avocado oil and spices. Spread the chicken and vegetables on the parchment-lined baking pan.

3. Spread the parmesan cheese on top, and cook in the oven for 15 minutes.

4. Remove the pan from the oven, and toss all the ingredients.

5. Top the chicken and vegetables with additional parmesan cheese, if desired, and cook for another 10 minutes or until the chicken reaches 165°F.

Calories: 395, **Protein:** 26 grams, **Carbohydrates:** 26 grams, **Fat:** 21 grams

Sheet-Pan Chicken Curry

This delicious sheet-pan dish is one of my favorite go-to dinners. It's a hearty chicken dinner that's perfect for busy weekday nights. It's delicious served over basmati or cauliflower rice.

Serves: 4 | **Prep/Cook Time:** 45 minutes

1½ pounds chicken breasts
1 (13.5-ounce) canned coconut milk
2 cups diced broccoli
2 cups diced cauliflower

1 red bell pepper, cut into large chunks
2 tablespoons curry powder
1 tablespoon lime juice
¼ teaspoon ginger powder

¼ teaspoon sea salt
⅛ teaspoon black pepper

fresh cilantro (optional)

1. Preheat the oven to 400°F.

2. Add all the ingredients to a 9x13-inch baking pan. Mix well.

3. Cook the mixture in the oven for 40 minutes, tossing the ingredients halfway through.

4. Remove the pan from the oven once the chicken reaches 165°F and the vegetables are tender.

5. Top with fresh cilantro if desired.

Calories: 360, **Protein:** 39 grams, **Carbohydrates:** 13 grams, **Fat:** 16 grams

Shrimp and Cabbage Bowls

These shrimp and cabbage bowls are a great combination of protein and gut-friendly ingredients!

Serves: 5–6 | **Prep/Cook Time:** 30 minutes

3 cups cooked brown rice
2 pounds shrimp
2 tablespoons avocado oil
2 tablespoons fresh lime juice
2 teaspoons ground cumin
1 teaspoon garlic powder

½ teaspoon sea salt
½ teaspoon black pepper
2 bags coleslaw mix
½ cup fresh chopped cilantro
Toppings: sesame seeds and avocado slices (optional)

1. Cook the rice according to its package directions.

2. Meanwhile, in a large bowl, marinate the shrimp with the avocado oil, lime juice, and spices in a large bag or container. Place the shrimp in the refrigerator for 20 minutes.

3. Remove the shrimp, add them to a large pan, and sauté them until the internal temperature reaches 145°F.

4. Add the coleslaw mixture and cilantro to the pan, and cook for an additional 5 minutes, or until the coleslaw is cooked down.

5. Serve the shrimp and coleslaw mixture over cooked rice and, if desired, top it with additional cilantro, avocado, and sesame seeds.

Calories: 332, **Protein:** 20 grams, **Carbohydrates:** 53 grams, **Fat:** 7 grams

Turkey Taco Casserole

This is a simple one-skillet taco dish that's packed with flavor. It makes great leftovers and can easily be frozen for later use.

Serves: 6 | Prep/Cook Time: 60 minutes

1 pound ground turkey
1 bell pepper, diced
2 cups spinach
1 onion, diced
2 teaspoons ground cumin
1 teaspoon garlic powder
½ teaspoon chili powder
1 (16-ounce) can salsa

1 (13-ounce) can black beans, rinsed and drained
2 cups water
1 cup brown rice
1 tablespoon lime juice
1 cup shredded cheese
Toppings: plain Greek yogurt, avocado, cilantro, or olives (optional)

1. Preheat the oven to 375°F.

2. In a large pan, cook the ground turkey until it's no longer pink.

3. Add the bell pepper, spinach, and onion, and sauté them for 5 minutes. Add in spices.

4. Pour the turkey and vegetables into a 9x13 pan. Add the salsa, black beans, water, brown rice, and lime juice.

5. Top everything with shredded cheese, and cover the pan with foil.

6. Cook in the oven for 60 minutes.

7. Remove the foil and let it cook for 10 minutes to thicken.

Calories: 395, **Protein:** 26 grams, **Carbohydrates:** 43 grams, **Fat:** 13 grams

Veggie Spaghetti Bake

Here's a veggie-loaded twist to your typical spaghetti meal! This is a one-pan dish that's perfect for busy nights.

Serves: 6 | Prep/Cook Time: 35 minutes

1 pound ground beef

3 cups diced zucchini

2 cups diced spinach

1 onion, diced

1 (24-ounce) jar spaghetti sauce (look for no sugar added)

1 cup water

1 (6-ounce) package chickpea penne pasta

½ tablespoon Italian seasoning

½ tablespoon garlic powder

½ teaspoon black pepper

½ teaspoon sea salt

1 cup parmesan cheese, for topping

1. Preheat the oven to 375°F.

2. Cook the beef in a medium-sized pan until it's no longer pink.

3. Add the beef along with the vegetables to a 9x13-inch baking pan.

4. Mix in the spaghetti sauce, water, chickpea noodles, and seasonings. Add the parmesan cheese on top of everything.

5. Cover the mixture with foil, and cook it in the oven for 30 minutes.

6. Remove the veggie spaghetti bake from the oven, and let it cool for 10 minutes to allow the sauce to thicken.

Calories: 356, **Protein:** 29 grams, **Carbohydrates:** 50 grams, **Fat:** 9 grams

SALADS

Cucumber, Tomato, and Feta Salad

This is a light and refreshing Greek salad that takes minutes to make using fresh ingredients. I love using this as a side dish or for lunch when paired with a protein like chicken.

Serves: 4 | Prep/Cook Time: 10 minutes

1 small English cucumber, diced
10 ounces cherry tomatoes, diced
½ cup chickpeas, rinsed and drained
½ cup feta
¼ cup fresh chopped cilantro

2 tablespoons extra-virgin olive oil
1 tablespoon minced garlic
1 tablespoon apple cider vinegar
½ teaspoon sea salt
½ teaspoon black pepper

1. Mix all the ingredients until well combined.

2. Serve cold and store in the refrigerator for up to three days.

Calories: 231, **Protein:** 8 grams, **Carbohydrates:** 27 grams, **Fat:** 11 grams

Dill and Cucumber Chicken Salad

If you're a fan of dill, you'll love this cucumber dill chicken salad. Serve it as a dip with veggies and crackers, in a wrap, or over some salad greens.

Serves: 4 | Prep/Cook Time: 5 minutes

1 pound cooked chicken, diced
¾ cup diced cucumbers
½ onion, diced
½ cup avocado-oil-based mayonnaise
½ cup plain Greek yogurt

1 tablespoon lemon juice
1 tablespoon dried dill
⅛ teaspoon black pepper
⅛ teaspoon sea salt

1. In a large bowl, mix all the ingredients until they're well combined.

2. Store this salad in an airtight container in the fridge for up to five days.

Calories: 211, **Protein:** 20 grams, **Carbohydrates:** 5 grams, **Fat:** 12.5 grams

Note: Make this dairy-free by replacing the Greek yogurt with mayonnaise.

Easy Egg Salad

This is an easy protein option that can be used as a dip with vegetables and crackers, in a wrap or sandwich, or over salad greens.

Serves: 3 | **Prep/Cook Time:** 10 minutes

6 hard-boiled eggs, chopped

¼ cup avocado-oil-based mayonnaise

¼ cup plain Greek yogurt

½ red bell pepper, chopped

2 tablespoons chopped green onions

1 teaspoon dijon mustard

1 teaspoon garlic powder

⅛ teaspoon paprika

⅛ teaspoon black pepper

⅛ teaspoon sea salt

1. Place the chopped eggs, mayonnaise, Greek yogurt, red bell peppers, green onion, and dijon mustard together in a bowl. Mix well. Season the mixture with the spices.

2. Serve this salad cold, and store it in the refrigerator for up to five days.

Note: You can replace all the mayonnaise for plain Greek yogurt for extra protein, or replace the Greek yogurt with mayonnaise to make it dairy-free.

Calories: 173, **Protein:** 18 grams, **Carbohydrates:** 5 grams, **Fat:** 17 grams

Kale and Apple Salad with Vinaigrette

Here's a fall-inspired salad with a crunch! This is the perfect combination of greens with sweetness.

Serves: 3–4 | **Prep/Cook Time:** 10 minutes

Salad

6 cups chopped kale

1 large red apple, diced

¼ cup chopped pecans

2 ounces goat cheese

Dressing

3 tablespoons extra-virgin olive oil

1½ tablespoons apple cider vinegar

2 teaspoons dijon mustard

1 teaspoon honey

1. In a large bowl, mix all the ingredients for the salad. Set it aside.

2. In a mason jar, add all the dressing ingredients. Mix well.

3. Pour the dressing over the salad, or serve it on the side.

Calories: 379, **Protein:** 6 grams, **Carbohydrates:** 40 grams, **Fat:** 18 grams

Lemon Pepper Salmon Salad

An easy protein salad that takes five minutes to make. Serve it over salad greens, in a wrap, or as a dip with vegetables and crackers.

Serves: 4 | **Prep/Cook Time:** 10 minutes

Salad

2 (6-ounce) cans wild-caught salmon

⅓ cup avocado-oil based mayonnaise

½ cup diced celery

½ onion, diced

½ tablespoon lemon pepper

1. In a large bowl, mix all the ingredients for the salad.

2. Serve this salad cold, and store it in the refrigerator for up to 5 days.

Calories: 206, **Protein:** 18 grams, **Carbohydrates:** 4 grams, **Fat:** 12 grams

Strawberry Goat Cheese Salad with Balsamic Vinaigrette

This is a refreshing salad topped with a touch of sweetness and made with a homemade balsamic vinaigrette. Serve it as a side salad, or pair it with a protein to make it a complete meal.

Serves: 4 | **Prep/Cook Time:** 10 minutes

Salad

8 cups loosely packed salad greens

2 cups diced strawberries

4 ounces plain goat cheese

2 tablespoons sunflower seeds

Balsamic Vinaigrette

½ cup extra-virgin olive oil

2 tablespoons balsamic vinegar

1 tablespoon dijon mustard

1 tablespoon minced garlic

1 teaspoon honey

1. In a large bowl, mix all the ingredients for the salad. Set it aside.

2. In a mason jar, add all the ingredients for the dressing. Mix well.

3. Pour the dressing over the salad, or serve it on the side.

Calories: 387, **Protein:** 7 grams, **Carbohydrates:** 23 grams, **Fat:** 35 grams

Thai Crunch Salad with Peanut Dressing

This Thai-inspired salad is made with a delicious peanut dressing. It's perfect for a side dish or as a balanced meal when topped with a protein like hard-boiled eggs, salmon, or chicken.

Serves: 4 | **Prep/Cook Time:** 10 minutes

Salad

6 cups loosely packed salad greens

1 bag coleslaw mix

½ cup loosely packed cilantro, chopped

1 cup peanuts, for topping

Peanut Dressing

¼ cup natural peanut butter

¼ cup water

3 tablespoons rice vinegar

3 tablespoons extra-virgin olive oil

2 tablespoons coconut aminos

2 teaspoons minced garlic

1. Place all the salad ingredients, except the peanuts, in a large bowl. Set it aside.

2. Mix the peanut dressing ingredients in a bowl, or shake them together in a mason jar.

3. Pour the dressing over the salad before serving, and top with peanuts.

Calories: 337, **Protein:** 13 grams, **Carbohydrates:** 19 grams, **Fat:** 25 grams

SIDES AND SNACKS

Almond Butter Bars

This is a no-bake protein bar that's filled with fiber, protein, and sweetness!

Makes: 6 bars | **Prep/Cook Time:** 1 hour, 5 minutes

1¼ cups rolled oats
½ cup vanilla protein powder
½ cup natural almond butter

⅓ cup maple syrup
1 tablespoon hemp seeds

1. Line a 9x5-inch baking dish with parchment paper.

2. Add all the ingredients in a medium bowl until they're well combined.

3. Next, press the mixture into the baking dish, and place it in the freezer for about one hour to set.

4. Remove the dish from the freezer, and cut the set mixture into 6 bars.

5. Store the bars in an airtight container in the freezer, and take them out as needed.

Calories: 199, **Protein:** 11 grams, **Carbohydrates:** 22 grams, **Fat:** 8 grams

Apple Cinnamon Cottage Cheese

This simple snack is made with just three ingredients that tastes like apple pie!

Serves: 1 | **Prep/Cook Time:** 5 minutes

½ cup cottage cheese
½ red apple, diced

⅛ teaspoon cinnamon

1. Mix all the ingredients together until well combined.

Calories: 160, **Protein:** 16 grams, **Carbohydrates:** 20 grams, **Fat:** 2 grams

Berry Almond Muffins

Here's a fiber-packed muffin loaded with blueberries without a lot of added sugar. Pair it with a protein to make it a balanced snack.

Makes: 12 muffins | **Prep/Cook Time:** 30 minutes

1 cup rolled oats

1 cup almond flour

1 tablespoon ground flaxseed

1 teaspoon baking soda

1 teaspoon cinnamon

¼ teaspoon sea salt

2 eggs

½ cup unsweetened almond milk

¼ cup maple syrup

1 teaspoon vanilla extract

1½ cups fresh blueberries

slivered almonds for topping

1. Preheat the oven to 350°F and line a muffin pan with muffin liners.

2. In a medium bowl, mix the oats, almond flour, flaxseed, baking soda, cinnamon, and sea salt.

3. In another bowl, mix together the eggs, almond milk, maple syrup, and vanilla until well combined. Pour the wet mixture into the dry ingredients.

4. Toss in the fresh blueberries.

5. Using an ice cream scooper, pour the batter into each individual muffin tin until about ¾ full.

6. Add slivered almonds on top of each muffin.

7. Bake the muffins in the oven for 25 minutes or until a toothpick inserted into the center of the muffin comes out clean.

(Per 1 muffin) Calories: 182, **Protein:** 6 grams, **Carbohydrates:** 20 grams, **Fat:** 7 grams

Chocolate Chia Seed Pudding

This six-ingredient chia seed pudding has 11 grams of fiber and makes a delicious snack or dessert.

Serves: 4 | **Prep/Cook Time:** 8 hours, 5 minutes

1⅓ cups milk of choice

½ cup chia seeds

¼ cup unsweetened cocoa powder

¼ cup maple syrup

| 1 teaspoon cinnamon | Toppings: whipped cream, raspberries, |
| ½ teaspoon vanilla extract | bananas, or strawberries (optional) |

1. In a medium bowl, whisk together all the ingredients until smooth.

2. Place bowl in the refrigerator for at least 3 hours.

3. Divide it into four servings, and add toppings if desired.

Calories: 254, **Protein:** 8 grams, **Carbohydrates:** 33 grams, **Fat:** 12 grams

Chocolate Chip Peanut Butter Bars

This no-bake bar is full of fiber, protein, and sweetness! Each bar contains 11 grams of protein, making it a great balanced option for a snack.

Makes: 6 bars | **Prep/Cook Time:** 1 hour, 5 minutes

1 cup natural peanut butter	1 tablespoon chia seeds
⅓ cup coconut flour	1 teaspoon vanilla extract
¼ cup collagen peptides powder	¼ teaspoon sea salt
2 tablespoons honey or maple syrup	½ cup dark chocolate chips

1. In a medium bowl, mix together all the ingredients, except the chocolate chips, until well combined.

2. Line a 9x5-inch baking dish (or something similar) with parchment paper. Evenly press the mixture down throughout the entire dish.

3. Sprinkle the chocolate chips on top (it helps to press the chocolate chips down into the mixture).

4. Place the bars in the freezer for about 1 hour to allow them to set.

5. Remove the set mixture from the freezer, and cut it into 6 bars.

6. Store the bars in the freezer and take them out as needed.

Calories: 261, **Protein:** 11 grams, **Carbohydrates:** 22 grams, **Fat:** 12 grams

Everything But the Bagel Veggie Dip

This is a simple dip that's delicious when it's paired with raw vegetables and served as a snack or appetizer.

Makes: 1 cup | **Prep/Cook Time:** 5 minutes

1 cup cottage cheese
½ cup plain Greek yogurt

1½ tablespoons everything
bagel seasoning

1. Mix all the ingredients together in a blender until smooth.

2. Serve the dip with veggies like carrots, cucumbers, or peppers.

(**Per ¼ cup**) **Calories:** 32, **Protein:** 5 grams, **Carbohydrates:** 1 gram, **Fat:** 1 gram

Trail Mix Peanut Butter Balls

These are sweet and salty bite-sized protein balls that make a great snack on the go!

Makes: 12–14 balls | **Prep/Cook Time:** 1 hour, 5 minutes

1 cup rolled oats
¾ cup trail mix (or a combination of peanuts, dried fruit, and seeds)
¼ cup ground flaxseed
1 teaspoon cinnamon

½ cup natural peanut butter
(or other nut butter)
¼ cup honey
½ teaspoon vanilla extract

1. Mix the oats, trail mix, flaxseed, and cinnamon together in a medium bowl.

2. Add in the peanut butter, honey, and vanilla extract. Mix all the ingredients well.

3. Roll the mixture into 1½-inch balls.

4. Place the balls on a plate, and put them in the freezer for one hour.

5. Remove the balls from the freezer, and store them in an airtight container in the refrigerator.

(**Per 1 ball**) **Calories:** 129, **Protein:** 4 grams,
Carbohydrates: 17 grams, **Fat:** 5 grams

Tuna Cucumber Bites

These bite-sized tuna cucumber bites are a great high-protein snack with a crunch.

Makes: 10 cucumber bites | **Prep/Cook Time:** 5 minutes

1 (5-ounce) can tuna packed in water

2 tablespoons avocado-oil-based mayonnaise

¼ teaspoon garlic powder

¼ teaspoon onion powder

⅛ teaspoon black pepper

⅛ teaspoon sea salt

1 medium English cucumber, cut into ten ½-inch slices

paprika, for topping

1. Mix the tuna, mayonnaise, garlic, onion, black pepper, and sea salt together in a bowl. Set the mixture aside.

2. Using a melon baller or spoon, scoop out the center of each cucumber. Set them on a plate.

3. Spoon the tuna mixture into each cucumber. Top each cucumber with paprika.

(Per 1 bite) Calories: 66, **Protein:** 7 grams, **Carbohydrates:** 4 grams, **Fat:** 2 grams

Yogurt Fruit Dip

This easy yogurt dip takes 5 minutes to make and is delicious when served with fruit like berries and apples.

Makes: 1 cup | **Prep/Cook Time:** 5 minutes

1 cup plain Greek yogurt

1 tablespoon maple syrup

1 teaspoon vanilla extract

1 teaspoon ground flaxseed or chia seeds

1. Mix all the ingredients together until well combined.

2. Serve the dip with fresh fruit.

(Per ¼ cup) Calories: 212, **Protein:** 7 grams, **Carbohydrates:** 24 grams, **Fat:** 8 grams

BEVERAGES

Coconut Lemon Mineral Mocktail

Here's a refreshing mocktail that takes minutes to make. I love having this first thing in the morning or in the afternoon for extra hydration.

Serves: 1 | **Prep/Cook Time:** 5 minutes

8 ounces unsweetened coconut water

lemon juice from ½ lemon

⅛ teaspoon sea salt

200 milligrams magnesium powder

ice

1. Mix all the ingredients together, and serve over ice.

> **Calories:** 52, **Protein:** 1 gram, **Carbohydrates:** 10 grams, **Fat:** 0.5 grams

Iced Coconut Matcha Latte

Matcha is a good source of L-theanine, an amino acid helpful for reducing stress. It also provides antioxidants and nutrients supportive for blood sugar.

Serves: 1 | **Prep/Cook Time:** 20 minutes

2 teaspoons matcha powder

1 cup, plus 2 teaspoons hot water

1 to 2 teaspoons maple syrup

1 teaspoon vanilla extract

ice cubes

⅓ cup coconut milk (from a can)

1. Mix together the matcha powder with 2 teaspoons of hot water until well combined. Pour in the remaining water, maple syrup, and vanilla extract.

2. Place the mixture in the refrigerator for 15 minutes to cool down.

3. Place the ice cubes in a 16-ounce glass.

4. Pour the matcha mixture into the glass, and pour the coconut milk on top. Mix well.

> **Calories:** 87, **Protein:** 1 gram, **Carbohydrates:** 18 grams, **Fat:** 2 grams

Immunity Tea

This is an antioxidant-packed tea to support a healthy immune system. I always make this when I'm not feeling well or need some extra gut support.

Makes: 1 cup | **Prep/Cook Time:** 5 minutes

1 cup green tea

1 teaspoon raw honey (local is best)

1 teaspoon apple cider vinegar

½ teaspoon cinnamon

juice from 1 lemon wedge (about 1 teaspoon)

1. Mix together all the ingredients and serve warm.

Calories: 27, **Protein:** 0.1 gram, **Carbohydrates:** 7 grams, **Fat:** 0.1 gram

Strawberry Lime Mineral Mocktail

This is refreshing mineral mocktail that takes minutes to make.

Serves: 1 | **Prep/Cook Time:** 5 minutes

8 ounces unsweetened coconut water

½ cup strawberry sparkling water

juice from ½ lime

200 milligrams magnesium powder

⅛ teaspoon sea salt

ice

1. Mix all the ingredients together. Serve over ice.

Calories: 52, **Protein:** 1 gram, **Carbohydrates:** 10 grams, **Fat:** 0.5 grams

Tropical Mineral Slushie

This is a summer-inspired beverage that tastes like a piña colada packed with minerals!

Serves: 1 | **Prep/Cook Time:** 5 minutes

1 cup frozen pineapple

½ cup unsweetened coconut water

1 tablespoon lime juice

200 milligrams magnesium powder

⅛ teaspoon sea salt

1. Place all the ingredients in a blender, and blend until smooth.

Calories: 152, **Protein:** 2 grams, **Carbohydrates:** 36 grams, **Fat:** 2 grams

Turmeric Golden Milk

Turmeric is a spice full of flavor and antioxidants. This golden milk makes a perfect beverage for a cold day, or when you want to boost your immunity.

Makes: 1 cup | **Prep/Cook Time:** 5 minutes

1 cup milk of choice

1 to 2 teaspoons maple syrup

½ teaspoon turmeric spice

½ teaspoon ground ginger

½ teaspoon cinnamon

½ teaspoon vanilla extract

pinch of ground black pepper
(helps with turmeric absorption)

1. Put all the ingredients into a saucepan and simmer (don't boil) for 10 minutes, or until warm.

Calories: 166, **Protein:** 8 grams, **Carbohydrates:** 16 grams, **Fat:** 8 grams

BIBLIOGRAPHY

CHAPTER 1

American Diabetes Association. "Statistics About Diabetes." Last updated November 2, 2023. https://diabetes.org/about-diabetes/statistics/about-diabetes.

CHAPTER 2

"Diabetes and Your Heart." *CDC.gov*. Last updated June 20, 2022. https://www.cdc .gov/diabetes/library/features/diabetes-and-heart.html

Kong, De-Xian, Yan-xin Xiao, Zhen-Xi-Zhang, and Ya-Bin Liu. "Study on the Correlation Between Metabolism, Insulin Sensitivity, and Progressive Weight Loss Change in Type-2 Diabetes." *Pakistan Journal of Medical Sciences* 36, no. 7 (2020). https://doi.org/10.12669/pjms.36.7.3027.

Manoogian, Emily N. C., Amandine Chaix, and Satchidananda Panda. "When to Eat: The Importance of Eating Patterns in Health and Disease." *Journal of Biological Rhythms* 34, no. 6 (2018). https://doi.org/10.1177/0748730419892105.

Tohru Hira, Trakooncharoenvit Aphichat, and Taguchi Hayate. "Improvement of Glucose Tolerance by Food Factors Having Glucagon-Like Peptide-1 Releasing Activity." *International Journal of Molecular Sciences* (2021). https://doi .org/10.3390/ijms22126623

CHAPTER 3

"The A1C Test & Diabetes." National Institutes of Health. Last updated April 2018. https://www.niddk.nih.gov/health-information/diagnostic-tests/a1c-test.

CHAPTER 4

Basturk, Berrak, Zeynep Koc Ozerson, and Aysun Yuksel. "Evaluation of the Effect of Macronutrients Combination on Blood Sugar Levels in Healthy Individuals." *Iran Journal of Public Health* (2021). https://doi.org/10.18502/ijph.v50i2.5340.

Blüher, Matthias. "Metabolically Healthy Obesity." *Endocrine Reviews* 41, no. 3 (2020). https://doi.org/10.1210/endrev/bnaa004.

"Chronic Diseases in America." CDC.gov. Last updated May 15, 2024. https://www .cdc.gov/chronic-disease/about/index.html.

"US Obesity Rates Have Tripled Over the Last 60 Years." USAFacts.org. Last updated March 21, 2023. https://usafacts.org/articles/obesity-rate-nearly -triples-united-states-over-last-50-years.

"Weight Loss Services in the US–Market Size (2003–2029)." IBISWorld.com. Last
   updated March 2, 2023. https://www.ibisworld.com/industry-statistics/market
   -size/weight-loss-services-united-states.

CHAPTER 5

Cava, Edda, Nai Chien Yeat, and Bettina Mittendorfer." Preserving Healthy Muscle
   During Weight Loss." *Advanced Nutrition* 8, no. 3. https://doi.org/10.3945
   /an.116.014506.

Chang, Chia-Yu, Der-Shin Ke, and Jen-Yin Chen. "Essential Fatty Acids and Human
   Brain." *Acta Neurologica Taiwanica* 18, no. 4 (2009): 231–41. https://pubmed
   .ncbi.nlm.nih.gov/20329590.

DiNicolantonio, James, and James O'Keefe. "The Importance of Maintaining a
   Low Omega-6/Omega-3 Ratio for Reducing the Risk of Autoimmune Diseases,
   Asthma, and Allergies." *Mo Med* 118, no. 5 (2021). https://www.ncbi.nlm.nih.gov
   /pmc/articles/PMC8504498.

Ghada, Soliman. "Dietary Cholesterol and the Lack of Evidence in Cardiovascular
   Disease." *Nutrients* 10, no. 6 (2018). https://doi.org/10.3390/nu10060780.

Ginter, E., and V. Simko. "New Data on Harmful Effects of Trans-Fatty Acids."
   Bratislava Medical Journal 117, no. 5 (2017). https://doi.org/10.4149
   /bll_2016_048.

Holesh, Julie, Sanah Aslam, and Andrew Martin. Physiology, Carbohydrates.
   Treasure Island, FL: StatPearls Publishing (2023). https://pubmed.ncbi.nlm.nih
   .gov/29083823.

Klemm, Sarah. "4 Keys to Strength Building and Muscle Mass." EatRight.org. Last
   updated January 21, 2021. https://www.eatright.org/fitness/physical-activity
   /benefits-of-exercise/4-keys-to-strength-building-and-muscle-mass.

Lacovides, Stella, Shane Maloney, Sindeep Bhana, Zareena Angamia, and Rebecca
   Meiring. "Could the Ketogenic Diet Induce a Shift in Thyroid Function and
   Support a Metabolic Advantage in Healthy Participants? A Pilot Randomized
   -Controlled-Crossover Trial." *PLOS ONE* 18, no. 11 (2023). https://doi.
   org/10.1371/journal.pone.0269440.

Moon, Jaecheol, and Gwanpyo Koh. "Clinical Evidence and Mechanisms of High
   -Protein Diet-Induced Weight Loss." *Journal of Obesity & Metabolic Syndrome*
   29, no.3 (2020). https://doi.org/10.7570/jomes20028.

"Most Heart Attack Patients' Cholesterol Levels Did Not Indicate Cardiac Risk."
   Science Daily. January 13, 2009. https://www.sciencedaily.com
   /releases/2009/01/090112130653.htm.

"Nutrition: Trans Fat." *World Health Organization.* May 3, 2018. https://www.who
   .int/news-room/questions-and-answers/item/nutrition-trans-fat.

"Omega-3 Fatty Acids." National Institutes of Health. July 18, 2022. https://ods
   .od.nih.gov/factsheets/Omega3FattyAcids-Consumer.

Pesta, Dominik H., and Samuel Varman. "A High-Protein Diet for Reducing Body Fat: Mechanisms and Possible Caveats." *Nutrition and Metabolism* 11, no. 53 (2014). https://doi.org/10.1186/1743-7075-11-53.

Qian, Frank, Andres Korat, Vasanti Malik, and Frank Hu. "Metabolic Effects of Monounsaturated Fatty Acid–Enriched Diets Compared with Carbohydrate or Polyunsaturated Fatty Acid–Enriched Diets in Patients with Type 2 Diabetes: A Systematic Review and Meta-analysis of Randomized Controlled Trials." *Diabetes Care* 39, no. 8 (2016). https://doi.org/10.2337/dc16-0513.

Radzikowska, Urszula Radzikowska, et al. "The Influence of Dietary Fatty Acids on Immune Responses." *Nutrients* 11, no, 12 (2019). https://doi.org/10.3390/nu11122990.

Sergin, Selin, Vijayashree Jambunathan, Esha Garg, Jason Rowntree, and Jenifer Fenton. "Fatty Acid and Antioxidant Profile of Eggs from Pasture-Raised Hens Fed a Corn- and Soy-Free Diet and Supplemented with Grass-Fed Beef Suet and Liver." *Foods* 11, no. 21 (2022). https://doi.org/10.3390/foods11213404.

Seungyoun, Jung, Olga Goloubeva, Erin LeBlanc, Linda Snetselaar, Linda Horn, and Joanne Dorgan. "Dietary Fat Intake During Adolescence and Breast Density Among Young Women." *Cancer Epidemiology, Biomarkers & Prevention* 25, no. 6 (2016). https://doi.org/10.1158/1055-9965.EPI-15-1146.

Siri-Tarino, Patty, Qi Sun, Frank Hu, and Ronald Krauss. "Meta-Analysis of Prospective Cohort Studies Evaluating the Association of Saturated Fat with Cardiovascular Disease." *The American Journal of Clinical Nutrition* 39, no. 8 (2016). https://doi.org/10.3945/ajcn.2009.27725.

"Small Entity Compliance Guide: Trans Fatty Acids in Nutrition Labeling, Nutrient Content Claims, and Health Claims." *FDA.* August 2003. https://www.fda.gov/regulatory-information/search-fda-guidance-documents/small-entity-compliance-guide-trans-fatty-acids-nutrition-labeling-nutrient-content-claims-and.

"Weighing in on Dietary Fats." National Institutes of Health. December 2011. https://newsinhealth.nih.gov/2011/12/weighing-dietary-fats.

Willet, Walter, and Rudolph Leibel. "Dietary Fat Is Not a Major Determinant of Body Fat." *American Journal of Medicine,* no. 113 (2002). https://doi.org/10.1016/s0002-9343(01)00992-5.

Xue, C., et al. "Consumption of Medium-and Long-Chain Triacylglycerols Decreases Body Fat and Blood Triglyceride in Chinese Hypertriglyceridemic Subjects." *European Journal of Clinical Nutrition* 63 (2009). https://doi.org/10.1038/ejcn.2008.76.

CHAPTER 6

Barclay, Alan, et al. "Dietary Glycemic Index Labelling: A Global Perspective." *Nutrients* 13, no. 9 (2021). https://doi.org/10.3390/nu13093244.

Harvard Medical School. "Choosing Good Carbs with the Glycemic Index." Harvard .edu. November 1, 2012. https://www.health.harvard.edu/staying-healthy /choosing-good-carbs-with-the-glycemic-index.

Jenkins, David, et al. "Glycemic Index, Glycemic Load, and Cardiovascular Disease and Mortality." *The New England Journal of Medicine* 384, no. 14. (2021). https://doi.org/10.1056/NEJMoa2007123.

Zafar, Mohammad, et al. "Low-Glycemic Index Diets as an Intervention for Diabetes: A Systematic Review and Meta-Analysis." *The American Journal of Clinical Nutrition* 110, no. 4 (2019). https://doi.org/10.1093/ajcn/nqz149.

CHAPTER 7

Akpınar, Serife, Makbule Gezman, and Karadag. "Is Vitamin D Important in Anxiety or Depression? What Is the Truth?" *Current Nutrition Reports* 11, no. 4 (2022). https://doi.org/10.1007/s13668-022-00441-0.

Asbaghi, O., et al. "Effect of Vitamin E Intake on Glycemic Control and Insulin Resistance in Diabetic Patients: An Updated Systematic Review and Meta-Analysis of Randomized Controlled Trials." *Nutrition Journal* 22, no. 10 (2023). https://doi.org/10.1186/s12937-023-00840-1.

Barbosa de Carvalho, Gabrielli, et al. "Zinc's Role in the Glycemic Control of Patients with Type 2 Diabetes: A Systematic Review." *Biometals* 30 (2017). https://doi.org/10.1007/s10534-017-9996-y.

Chatterjee, Ranee, Hsin-Chieh Yeh, David Edelman, and Frederick Brancati. "Potassium and Risk of Type 2 Diabetes." *Expert Review of Endocrinology & Metabolism* 6, no. 5 (2011). https://doi.org/10.1586/eem.11.60.

Dakhale, Ganesh, Harshal Chaudhari, and Meena Shrivastava. "Supplementation of Vitamin C Reduces Blood Glucose and Improves Glycosylated Hemoglobin in Type 2 Diabetes Mellitus: A Randomized, Double-Blind Study." *Advances in Pharmacological and Pharmaceutical Sciences* 2011 (2011). https://doi .org/10.1155/2011/195271.

"Diet, Nutrition and Prevention of Chronic Diseases." *WHO Technical Report Series* 916 (2003). https://iris.who.int/bitstream/handle/10665/42665/WHO_TRS _916.pdf;jsessionid=7B82665C7D5C1187D313A8A5333359FF?sequence=1.

Ellison, Deborah, and Heather Moran. "Vitamin D: Vitamin or Hormone?" *Nursing Clinics of North America* 56, no. 1 (2021). https://doi.org/10.1016/j.cnur .2020.10.004.

"Folate." National Institutes of Health. November 2022. https://ods.od.nih.gov /factsheets/Folate-Consumer.

Pittas, Anastassios, Joseph Lau, Frank Hu, and Bess Dawson-Hughes. "The Role of Vitamin D and Calcium in Type 2 Diabetes. A Systematic Review and Meta-Analysis." *The Journal of Clinical Endocrinology & Metabolism* 92, no. 6 (2007). https://doi.org/10.1210/jc.2007-0298.

"Vitamin D." National Institutes of Health. September 2023. https://ods.od.nih.gov/factsheets/VitaminD-HealthProfessional.

"Vitamin E." National Institutes of Health. March 2021. https://ods.od.nih.gov/factsheets/VitaminE-HealthProfessional.

"Vitamins and Minerals for Older Adults." National Institutes of Health. January 2, 2021. https://www.nia.nih.gov/health/vitamins-and-supplements/vitamins-and-minerals-older-adults.

Weyh, Christopher, Karsten Krüger, Peter Peeling, and Lindy Castell. "The Role of Minerals in the Optimal Functioning of the Immune System." *Nutrients* 14, no. 3 (2022). https://doi.org/10.3390/nu14030644.

Zhao, Jie V., Mary Schooling, and Jia Xi Zhao. "The Effects of Folate Supplementation on Glucose Metabolism and Risk of Type 2 Diabetes: A Systematic Review and Meta-Analysis of Randomized Controlled Trials." *Annals of Epidemiology* 28, no. 4, https://doi.org/10.1016/j.annepidem.2018.02.001.

"Zinc." National Institutes of Health. September 2022. https://ods.od.nih.gov/factsheets/Zinc-HealthProfessional.

CHAPTER 8

"Added Sugar." *Harvard Health.* April 2022. https://www.hsph.harvard.edu/nutritionsource/carbohydrates/added-sugar-in-the-diet.

"Erythritol and Cardiovascular Events." National Institutes of Health. March 14, 2023. https://www.nih.gov/news-events/nih-research-matters/erythritol-cardiovascular-events.

Fagherazzi, Guy, et al. "Chronic Consumption of Artificial Sweetener in Packets or Tablets and Type 2 Diabetes Risk: Evidence from the E3N-European Prospective Investigation into Cancer and Nutrition Study." *Annals of Nutrition and Metabolism* 70, no. 1 (2017). https://doi.org/10.1159/000458769.

Pearlman, Michelle. "The Association Between Artificial Sweeteners and Obesity." *Current Gastroenterology Reports* 19, no. 64 (2017). https://doi.org/10.1007/s11894-017-0602-9.

Nettleton, Jodi, Raylene Reimer, and Jane Shearer. "Reshaping the Gut Microbiota: Impact of Low Calorie Sweeteners and the Link to Insulin Resistance?" *Physiology & Behavior* 164 (2016). https://doi.org/10.1016/j.physbeh.2016.04.029.

"The Nutrition Facts Label." *FDA.* 2023. The Nutrition Facts Label." FDA. 2023. https://www.fda.gov/food/nutrition-education-resources-materials/nutrition-facts-label.

"Types of Food Ingredients." *FDA*. Last updated July 6, 2023. https://www.fda.gov
/food/food-additives-and-gras-ingredients-information-consumers/types-food
-ingredients.

CHAPTER 9

Cahill, Leah, et al. "Prospective Study of Breakfast Eating and Incident Coronary
Heart Disease in a Cohort of Male US Health Professionals." *Circulation* 128,
no. 4 (2013). https://doi.org/10.1161/CIRCULATIONAHA.113.001474.

Collier, Roger. "Intermittent Fasting: The Science of Going Without." *Canadian
Medical Association Journal* 185, no. 9 (2013). https://doi.org/10.1503
/cmaj.109-4451.

Jakubowicz, Daniela, et al. "Fasting Until Noon Triggers Increased Postprandial
Hyperglycemia and Impaired Insulin Response After Lunch and Dinner in
Individuals with Type 2 Diabetes: A Randomized Clinical Trial." *Diabetes Care*
38, no. 10 (2015). https://doi.org/10.2337/dc15-0761.

Jakubowicz, Daniela, et al. "High Caloric Intake at Breakfast vs. Dinner
Differentially Influences Weight Loss of Overweight and Obese Women." *Obesity*
21, no. 12 (2013). https://doi.org/10.1002/oby.20460.

Marriam, Ali, et al. "Associations between Timing and Duration of Eating and
Glucose Metabolism: A Nationally Representative Study in the U.S." *Nutrients*
15, no. 3 (2023). https://doi.org/10.3390/nu15030729.

Takagi, Hisato, et al. "Meta-Analysis of Relation of Skipping Breakfast with Heart
Disease." *The American Journal of Cardiology* 124, no. 6 (2019). https://doi
.org/10.1016/j.amjcard.2019.06.016.

CHAPTER 10

"No More 'Clean Plate Club.'" HealthyChildren.org. Last updated March 27, 2014.
https://www.healthychildren.org/English/healthy-living/nutrition/Pages
/The-Clean-Plate-Club.aspx.

O'Reilly, G., et al. "Mindfulness-Based Interventions for Obesity-Related Eating
Behaviors: A Literature Review." *Obesity Reviews* 15, no. 6 (2014). https://doi
.org/10.1111/obr.12156.

CHAPTER 11

Dmitrieva, Natalia I., et al. "Middle-Age High Normal Serum Sodium as a Risk
Factor for Accelerated Biological Aging, Chronic Diseases, and Premature
Mortality." *EbioMedicine* 87 (2023). https://doi.org/10.1016/j.ebiom
.2022.104404.

Johnson, Evan, et al. "Reduced Water Intake Deteriorates Glucose Regulation in Patients with Type 2 Diabetes." *Nutrition Research* 43 (2017). https://doi.org/10.1016/j.nutres.2017.05.004.

Liska, DeAnn, et al. "Narrative Review of Hydration and Selected Health Outcomes in the General Population." *Nutrients* 11, no.1 (2019). https://doi.org/10.3390/nu11010070.

Riebel, Shaun, and Brenda Davy. "The Hydration Equation: Update on Water Balance and Cognitive Performance." *American College of Sports Medicine Health & Fitness Journal* 17, no. 6 (2013). https://doi.org/10.1249/FIT.0b013e3182a9570f.

Van Walleghen, Emily, et al. "Pre-meal Water Consumption Reduces Meal Energy Intake in Older but Not Younger Subjects." *Obesity* 15, no. 1 (2012). https://doi.org/10.1038/oby.2007.506.

Vij, Vinu, and Anjali Joshi. "Effect of 'Water Induced Thermogenesis' on Body Weight, Body Mass Index and Body Composition of Overweight Subjects." *Journal of Clinical and Diagnostic Research* 7, no. 9 (2013). https://doi.org/10.7860/JCDR/2013/5862.3344.

CHAPTER 14

Chan, Sharon, and Miguel Debono. "Replication of Cortisol Circadian Rhythm: New Advances in Hydrocortisone Replacement Therapy." *Therapeutic Advances in Endocrinology and Metabolism* 1, no. 3 (2010). https://doi.org/10.1177/2042018810380214.

Madison, Annelise, et al. "Omega-3 Supplementation and Stress Reactivity Of Cellular Aging Biomarkers: An Ancillary Substudy of a Randomized, Controlled Trial in Midlife Adults." *Mol Psychiatry* 26 (2021). https://doi.org/10.1038/s41380-021-01077-2.

Rosenkranz, Melissa, et al. "A Comparison of Mindfulness-Based Stress Reduction and an Active Control in Modulation of Neurogenic Inflammation." *Brain, Behavior, and Immunity* 27 (2013). https://doi.org/10.1016/j.bbi.2012.10.013.

"Stress and Sleep." *American Psychological Association.* Accessed April 23, 2024. https://www.apa.org/news/press/releases/stress/2013/sleep.

"Stress in America 2023." *American Psychological Association.* November 2023. https://www.apa.org/news/press/releases/stress/2023/collective-trauma-recovery.

"Vitamin C." National Institutes of Health. Last updated March 26, 2021. https://ods.od.nih.gov/factsheets/VitaminC-HealthProfessional.

"Workplace Stress." U.S. Department of Labor. Accessed April 23, 2024. https://www.osha.gov/workplace-stress.

CHAPTER 15

Aleman, Ricardo, et al. "Leaky Gut and the Ingredients That Help Treat It: A Review." *Molecules* 28, no. 2 (2023). https://doi.org/10.3390/molecules 28020619.

Berbudi, Afiat, et al. "Type 2 Diabetes and Its Impact on the Immune System." *Diabetes Reviews* 16, no. 5 (2020). https://doi.org/10.2174/1573399815666191 024085838.

Davis, Cindy. "The Gut Microbiome and Its Role in Obesity." *Nutrition* 51, no. 4 (2016). https://doi.org/10.1097/NT.0000000000000167.

"Digestive Diseases Statistics for the United States." National Institutes of Health. Last updated November 2014. https://www.niddk.nih.gov/health-information /diagnostic-tests/a1c-test.

Oana Iatcu, Camelia, et al. "Gut Microbiota and Complications of Type-2 Diabetes." *Nutrients* 14, no. 1 (2022). https://doi.org/10.3390/nu14010166.

Sadagopan, Aishwarya, et al. "Understanding the Role of the Gut Microbiome in Diabetes and Therapeutics Targeting Leaky Gut: A Systematic Review." *Cureus* 15, no. 7 (2023). https://doi.org/10.7759/cureus.41559.

Vanhaecke, Tiphaine, et al. "Drinking Water Source and Intake Are Associated with Distinct Gut Microbiota Signatures in US and UK Populations." *The Journal of Nutrition* 152, no. 1 (2022). https://doi.org/10.1093/jn/nxab312.

Willingham, Emily. "Some Sugar Substitutes Affect Blood Glucose and Gut Bacteria." *Scientific American.* August 19, 2022. https://www.scientificamerican. com/article/some-sugar-substitutes-affect-blood-glucose-and-gut-bacteria.

Yuanyuan, Li, et al. "The Role of Microbiome in Insomnia, Circadian Disturbance and Depression." *Front Psychiatry* 5, no. 9 (2018). https://doi.org/10.3389 /fpsyt.2018.00669.

CHAPTER 16

"Get Active!" *Centers for Disease Control and Prevention.* November 2022. https:// www.cdc.gov/diabetes/managing/active.html.

"How Much Physical Activity Do Adults Need?" Centers for Disease Control and Prevention. June 2022. https://www.cdc.gov/physicalactivity/basics/adults /index.htm.

Mathews, Charles, et al. "Amount of Time Spent in Sedentary Behaviors in the United States, 2003–2004." *American Journal of Epidemiology* 167, no. 7 (2008). https://doi.org/0.1093/aje/kwm390.

Momma, Haruki, et al. "Muscle-Strengthening Activities Are Associated with Lower Risk and Mortality in Major Non-Communicable Diseases: A Systematic Review and Meta-Analysis of Cohort Studies." *British Journal of Sports Medicine* 56, no. 13 (2022). https://bjsm.bmj.com/content/56/13/755.

CHAPTER 17

"Alcohol and Sleep." Sleep Foundation. January 2024. https://www.sleep foundation.org/nutrition/alcohol-and-sleep.

"Bedroom Environment: What Elements Are Important?" Sleep Foundation. March 2024. https://www.sleepfoundation.org/bedroom-environment.

"Waking Up at 4am Every Day? Here's Why." Sleep Foundation. January 2024. https://www.sleepfoundation.org/sleep-hygiene/why-do-i-wake-up-at-the -same-time-every-night.

"What Are Sleep Deprivation and Deficiency?" National Institutes of Health. March 2022. https://www.nhlbi.nih.gov/health/sleep-deprivation.

CHAPTER 18

Aljabri, Khalid, et al. "Glycemic Changes After Vitamin D Supplementation in Patients with Type 1 Diabetes Mellitus and Vitamin D Deficiency." *Annals of Saudi Medicine* 30, no. 6 (2010). https://doi.org/10.4103/0256-4947.72265.

Cao, Changfu, and Meiqing Su. "Effects Of Berberine on Glucose-Lipid Metabolism, Inflammatory Factors and Insulin Resistance in Patients with Metabolic Syndrome." *Experimental and Therapeutic Medicine* 17, no. 4 (2019). https://doi .org/10.3892/etm.2019.7295.

Capece, Umberto, et al. "Alpha-Lipoic Acid and Glucose Metabolism: A Comprehensive Update on Biochemical and Therapeutic Features." *Nutrients* 15, no. 1 (2022). https://doi.org/10.3390/nu15010018.

Dastgerdi, Azadehalsadat, et al. "The Therapeutic Effects of Magnesium in Insulin Secretion and Insulin Resistance." *Advanced Biomedical Research* 11, no. 54 (2022). https://doi.org/10.4103/abr.abr_366_21.

Havel, Peter. "A Scientific Review: The Role of Chromium in Insulin Resistance." *The Diabetes Educator* (2004). https://pubmed.ncbi.nlm.nih.gov/15208835.

Jin, Yinhli, et al. "Berberine Enhances the AMPK Activation and Autophagy and Mitigates High Glucose-Induced Apoptosis of Mouse Podocytes." *European Journal of Pharmacology* 5 (2017). https://doi.org/10.1016/j.ejphar.2016.11.037.

Lan, Jiarong, et al. "Meta-Analysis of the Effect and Safety of Berberine in the Treatment of Type 2 Diabetes Mellitus, Hyperlipemia and Hypertension." *Journal of Ethnopharmacology* (2015). https://doi.org/10.1016/j .jep.2014.09.049.

Lepretti, Marilena, et al. "Omega-3 Fatty Acids and Insulin Resistance: Focus on the Regulation of Mitochondria and Endoplasmic Reticulum Stress." *Nutrients* 10, no. 3 (2018). https://doi.org/10.3390/nu10030350.

ACKNOWLEDGMENTS

I've realized that writing a book is like raising a child. It's filled with love and excitement, and also a lot of patience and struggles. And just like raising a child, it takes a village. There are so many people that were involved in the creation of this book that I would like to thank.

First, thank you to everyone at Ulysses Press for being so wonderful to work with, especially Claire Sielaff. From editing the book to deciding on a book cover, you made my experience of writing a book so easy and encouraging. I cannot thank you all the hard work that went into bringing this book to fruition.

To my amazing husband, Kyle, who has always been my biggest supporter from day one. Thank you for all the times you took over things at home so I could have quiet time to write. I appreciate all you do and love you with all my heart.

To my children, Adelyn and Oliver, thank you for making me your mom. You are both the reason why I strive to be the best and healthiest version of myself. I appreciate all your encouragement, love, and recipe taste-testing. Especially when you would tell me, "Mom! This recipe is really good! It should be in your book!" I love you both so much.

To my parents, Ron and Dawn, thank you for always encouraging me to pursue my passion and helping to shape me into the person I am today.

To my grandma Delpha, thank you for your sweet soul, and always inspiring me to create something new in the kitchen.

To my sisters April and Amber, thank you for all the wisdom, laughter, and encouragement.

To the rest of my family, friends, teachers, and colleagues who have showed me so much support and encouragement throughout this whole journey. I cannot thank you enough.

To my amazing clients that I've had the privilege to serve for the past ten-plus years. Thank you for trusting me in your health journey, and teaching me so much about health. Your stories and successes are what shaped this book.

A huge thank you to my assistants Joyce and Eliza, who helped me keep my head above water while I was writing this. Thank you for all your hard work and continued support.

Lastly, thank you to you, the reader. Thank you for picking up this book in the first place and taking the initiative to learn and grow.

I love you all.

ABOUT THE AUTHOR

Autumn Enloe is an award-winning registered dietitian and writer from Minnesota. She's been writing for publications worldwide for over a decade and is passionate about empowering others to take control of their health through sustainable nutrition and lifestyle changes.

Autumn holds a master's degree in food and nutritional sciences and is the owner of Autumn Enloe Nutrition, a virtual private practice focused on optimizing metabolic and hormone health for women. She's on a mission to help others make healthy living their norm, and to create healthier generations to come.

Keep in touch with Autumn by visiting her website autumnenloe.com, and find her on Facebook and Instagram @autumn.enloe.nutrition.